T0152958

Youth Extension
A to Z

Dr. Beverly Potter

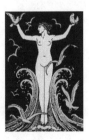

Ronin Publishng, Inc.
Berkeley, CA

Youth Extension A to Z

Copyright 2010: Beverly A. Potter
ISBN: 978-1-57951-090-9

Published by
Ronin Publishing, Inc.
PO Box 22900
Oakland, CA 94609
www.roninpub.com

All rights reserved. No part of this work may be reproduced or transmitted in any form by any means electronic or mechanical, including photocopying recording or translating into another language, or by any information storage or retrieval system, without written permission from the author or the publisher, except for inclusion of brief quotations in a review.

Fonts

Adobe Garamond—Adobe Systems

Dalliance—Emigre

Blown Deadline—Chank

Library of Congress Card Number: 2009913607
Distributed to the book trade by PGW/Perseus

NOTICE TO READER:
The material in this book is presented for educational purposes only. Publisher and author make no warranties about the validity or safety of the information provided. Reader should use due diligence in researching the material and applying to oneself. When in doubt, consult your health practitioner or other health care or mental health professional.

Youth Extension
A to Z

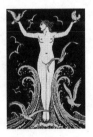

Dr. Beverly Potter

"Docpotter"

Other Books by Docpotter

Managing Yourself for Excellence
How to Become a Can-Do Person

Overcoming Job Burnout
How to Renew Enthusiasm for Work

The Worrywart's Companion
Twenty-One Ways to Soothe Yourself & Worry Smart

From Conflict to Cooperation
How to Mediate a Dispute

Finding a Path with a Heart
How to Go from Burnout to Bliss

Preventing Job Burnout
A Workbook

The Way of the Ronin
Riding the Waves of Change at Work

High Performance Goal Setting
Using Intuition to Conceive & Achieve Your Dreams

Beyond Conscious
What Happens After Death

Brain Boosters
Foods & Drugs that Make You Smarter

Drug Testing at Work
A Guide for Employers

Passing the Test
An Employee's Guide to Drug Testing

The Healing Magic of Cannabis
It's the High that Heals

Turning Around
Keys to Motivation and Productivity

Table of Contents

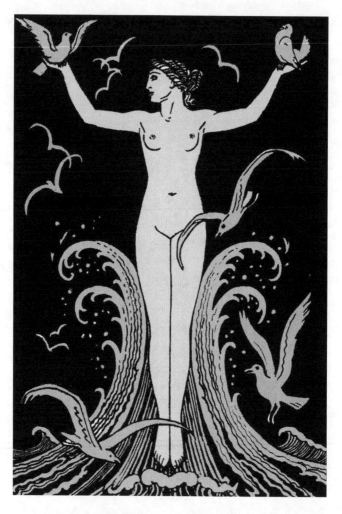

Youth is, after all, just a moment, but
it is the moment, the spark, that you
always carry in your heart.

—Raisa M. Gorbachev

What Is Youth Extension?

most of us want to live longer and want our senior years to be vibrant, healthy, active and youthful. Being youthful goes deeper than just appearing younger than one's actual years— it is not a matter of number of years lived. Youthful is somebody who has the characteristics of youth—good general health, strong muscles and bones, an efficient immune system, sharp memory, a healthy brain, and hormones working optimally.

We want to look good, with beautiful, glowing, youthful skin, the vitality we had in our twenties and thirties, and the capability to enjoy life to its fullest. *Youth Extension A to Z* is packed with ways to do so.

Today, people in their 60's, and well beyond, continue to push themselves physically and mentally to higher levels. They start businesses and climb mountains. For these folks youthful does not refer to age, but being lucid and agile, fully supportive and contributing to the community, enriching society with their vast range of experience and skills.

Growing old is inevitable; living old, however, is a choice. Physical aging is an un-avoidable reality. There is nothing that we can do to stop time from passing. We can, however, slow or speed

The worst enemy of life and health is the myth of aging!

—Walter Pierpaoli, M.D.
The Melatonin Miracle

up aging by our lifestyle and actions. Youth Extension is about living young, regardless of the number of years you have under you belt.

What is Youth?

Youth is that time between being a child and being an adult. Youth has a freshness and innocence. Words like vigor, flexibility, smooth body surfaces, natural, fertility, bloom, and spring suggest youth. Youth is fluid, rather than fixed. It is the absence of fixed decisions. It is changeable, impetuous, spontaneous, uninhibited, and risk-taking. Youth is playful, silly, and bouncy. It is a time filled with possibilities and dreams. Youth has unused store of energy, is unpiped and still ascending. Youth has a spirit of adventure, of joy, by a kind of impetuosity, often even by easily aroused enthusiasm, a carefree confidence, an exuberance that seems to indicate inexhaustible strength.

As an in-between time, youth is allowed considerable latitude to experiment and explore before entering the world of the mature. Most of us look back upon youth as a carefree time, while forgetting the stings and stumbles we suffered because hindsight is nostalgic.

By contrast, aging saps strength and ability to enjoy life. It cripples and eventually kills. To be "old" is someone who has succumbed to the problems related to age. Aging is the progressive failing ability of the body's intrinsic and genetic powers to defend, maintain, and repair itself in order to keep working efficiently. It is a declining body that has lost its strength and energy, so settled in a single groove as to be unable to turn without excessive difficulty, the mind becomes mechanized and rusty, slowed down and practically incapable of attending to any new ideas.

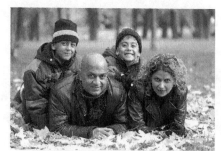

Youthfulness is a state of mind.

Do Not Go Gentle Into That Good Night

Do not go gentle into that good night,
Old age should burn and rave at close of day;
Rage, rage against the dying of the light.

Though wise men at their end know dark is right,
Because their words had forked no lightning they
Do not go gentle into that good night.

Good men, the last wave by, crying how bright
Their frail deeds might have danced in a green bay,
Rage, rage against the dying of the light.

Wild men who caught and sang the sun in flight,
And learn, too late, they grieved it on its way,
Do not go gentle into that good night.

Grave men, near death, who see with blinding sight
Blind eyes could blaze like meteors and be gay,
Rage, rage against the dying of the light.

And you, my father, there on the sad height,
Curse, bless, me now with your fierce tears, I pray.
Do not go gentle into that good night.
Rage, rage against the dying of the light.

— Dylan Thomas to his dying father

> **When it comes to staying young, a mind-lift beats a face-lift any day.**
>
> —Marty Bucella

As we grow older, we are subjected to an increasing number of external and internal damaging events, which are not being properly controlled, leading to illness and disability. Everything that obstructs, which uses up vital energies, that impoverishes or immobilizes, is tending towards old age.

Staying young while growing old begins with the mind. The old adage, "You're as young as you think" is surprisingly true, a kind of self-fulfilling prophecy because much of the way that we live comes from our mental attitude. Think young to live younger longer. Get in touch with your inner teenager. Greet each day, regardless of the weather, with wonder. Use your mind for constructive things, such as mentoring someone, doing volunteer work. Set a goal for each day. Clean the garbage out of your mind.

Exercise. Get in shape. Choose activities that you enjoy—perhaps bike riding, swimming, walking your dog. Join a fitness center and use it. Cultivate a youthful lifestyle. Be adaptive. Learn to accept change. Willingness to grow personally is a hallmark of one with a young outlook. Relaxing and maintaining a positive outlook in life is effective in combating aging. Stress accelerates aging. Unhealthy habits and laziness age you. Vices do not do you any good.

Being youthful lets you tap into new opportunities and embrace new ideas in life. Be eager to take on new challenges in daily life. Develop a positive outlook. Build up areas of your life that need development. Keep yourself looking good. Exercise for high energy, vitality and muscle strength. Continually improve your mind and intellect, add new skills to enrich life. Purposefully enjoy day-to-day life experience to plenty of enthusiasm to share with your family, children and grandchildren.

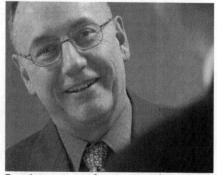

Staying young begins in the mind.

We were told that the brain continually loses cells and naturally dims with age but it turns out that this is a myth. Latest research reveals

Aging is inevitable; growing old is optional.

—Paul Bernstein
Mr. Physical Fitness USA™

that the brain is "plastic". That is, it is flexible and changing. "Use it or lose it" applies to the brain. When we continue to challenge our minds and stimulate our creativity, we not only feel better, we also cause our brains to sprout new branches, or dendrites. These new branches actually improve brain function and help compensate for the small loss of brain cells that does comes with age. In effect, the aging brain responds to mental exercise in much the same way that muscles responds to physical exercise.

Youth Extension A to Z explores the multitude of ways that you can extend youthfulness—a smorgasbord of possibilities to sample. Some you will already be doing, others will be new to you. You will resonate with some; others you'll pass by. This is a beginning, a launching of new possibilities, new horizons, a renewal of abundance and exuberance for living.

There is a fountain of youth: it is your mind, your talents, the creativity you bring to your life and the lives of people you love. When you learn to tap this source, you will truly have defeated age.

—Sophia Loren

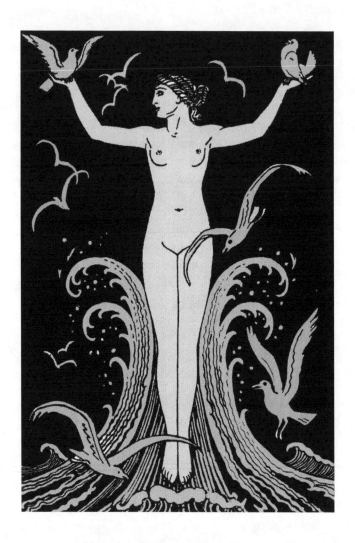

You can't help getting older,
but you don't have to get old.

~George Burns

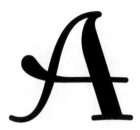

Acetyl-L-Carnitine

Acetyl-L-Carnitine is an amino acid that boosts mitochondrial energy production in the brain by facilitating fatty acid transport and oxidation in the cells. It slows effects of aging, decreases symptoms of depression. When taken as a supplement the mind-boosting effect is usually noticed within a few hours. Most people report feeling mentally sharper, having more focus and being more alert. Some find it to give a mild mood enhancement. Acetyl-L-Carnitine is found in red meats like beef and lamb, vegtables and grains.

Act As If

The first step in becoming a winner is to act like one. The same principle holds for being youthful—act as if you are young! The body follows where the mind leads. By "acting as if" you convince your mind that you already are what you want to become. Pretend just like you did when you were a kid. *Act youthful.*

Look for people who act youthful in the way that you would like to become. They may be friends, or even characters in novels or on

If you want a quality, act 'as if' you already have it.

—William James

television. Create an image in your mind of that person and how he or she behaves moment to moment—act as if you are already that person. Ask yourself would that person do right now? Then you do it. Acting as if keeps you focused on your desire. Soon you will no longer be acting, you will be being your youthful self.

Active Lifestyle

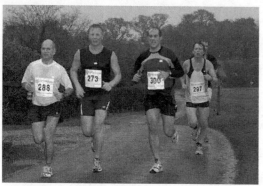

An active lifestyle keeps us youthful.

An active lifestyle leads to a better cardio functioning, faster metabolic rate, and faster burning of calories. Fit is fast, and effective. Just adding a little bit more effort in your physical activity will work as an anti-aging formula. Walking is one of the simplest ways to become more active. Take every opportunity that you can find to leave your car and walk. You will rejuvenate your bod and save the Earth, both!

Acupuncture

Acupuncture works directly with the body's energy or *qi* (pronounced chee). Acupuncture practitioners believe that all illnesses are a result of the natural flow of energy through the body becoming stuck, depleted or weakened and thus making the individual susceptible to illness. Best known for the control of pain, acupuncture has been effectively used for the treatment of back pain, headache, migraine, and sports injuries. It is helpful in treating anxiety, insomnia, digestive problems, abdominal, menstrual cramps, weight control, infertility.

Cosmetic acupuncture stimulates the circulation of *qi* to the face and neck, bringing blood and energy flow to the skin and the connective tissue beneath it—brightening and firming. Procedures can smooth fine lines, reduce the appearance of deeper wrinkles, plump out the texture of skin and help tone underlying muscles to tighten saggy cheeks and droopy necks.

Adventure

Adventure is an undertaking, often involving risk and danger, where you pit yourself against a significant challenge. It can be a wild and exciting pursuit, where you don't know what you will discover around the next bend. Adventure is state of mind—a playfulness and ability to build up suspense and to find wonder in small discoveries. The exhilaration of adventure is rejuvenating. Even small activities, like going on a Sunday drive, can be an adventure, finding delight in stopping at a roadside attraction or talking with a stranger. An adventuresome mind is a youthful mind.

Almond Facial Mask

Use crushed almonds in a facial mask. Grind almonds to a paste in the blender by mixing them with just enough olive oil to make blending easy. Rub the paste all over your face, allow to dry for fifteen minutes, and then wash off with warm water. Not only will healthful properties from the almonds soak into your skin, little bits of almond will exfoliate your skin, leaving it glowing, smooth, and youthful looking.

Aloe Vera

Aloe Vera is a natural vegetarian source of Vitamin B-12 and contains minerals vital to the growth process and healthy function of bodily systems. It acts as an antibacterial, antiviral and antifungal agent, preventing illness. The overall effect of taking Aloe Vera juice regularly can be a feeling of energy and health.

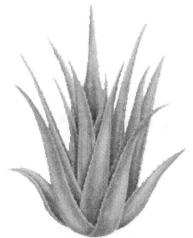

Aloe Vera is great for skin.

Aloe Vera juice is one of the finest body cleansers, cleaning morbid matter from the stomach, liver, kidneys, spleen, bladder, and is the finest, known colon cleanser. It relieves indigestion, stomach distress and ulcers. People claim relief from arthritis, bladder and kidney infections; leg cramps, constipation, hemorrhoids, and insomnia. It is an excellent general health tonic for energy and well-being.

Anti-Inflammatory Foods

Foods fit into three categories: pro-inflammatory, neutral, or anti-inflammatory. Aging at the cellular level can be slowed by eating anti-inflammatory foods that are rich in antioxidants, such as cold-water fish and richly colored fruits and vegetables. By contrast, eating foods classified as pro-inflammatory accelerates aging. Eating large amounts of saturated or trans-fatty acids, sugars, and starches causes insulin levels to surge and triggers an anti-inflammatory response that accelerates the aging process.

Antioxidants

Antioxidants protect cells from the ill-effects of oxidation called "free radicals". Vitamin E, C and A have strong antioxidant properties that reduce the risk of cardiovascular diseases and help slow aging. An antioxidant-rich diet can improve short-term memory, while slowing age-related decline in a variety of learning tasks. Foods rich in antioxidants include leafy greens like kale and spinach; vegetables including broccoli, beets, bell peppers, onions, garlic, cauliflower, and corn; as well as fruit like pomegranates, prunes, and most types of berries. Foods with color like blue or red, are high in antioxidants.

Aphrodisiacs

An aphrodisiac arouses or intensifies sexual desire. Yohimbe, Panax Ginseng, and Astralugus have been used to increase erotic desire for thousands of years. Aphrodisiacs work in several ways. They may directly increase the physical desire to have sex, stimulate the strength and endurance of an erection in men, and increase lubrication and genital sensitivity in women.

Aphrodisiacs for men work their magic in several ways. They can prolong and strengthen an erection and heighten the desire to have sex, enhance virility or can even be used to treat certain physiological conditions like sexual dysfunction and impotence. Feeling sexy is tremendously rejuvenating. Wow!

Apples

Remember the slogan, "An apple a day keeps the doctor away." Apples contain a flavonoid called quercetin that protects the brain from neurodegenerative diseases like Parkinson's and Alzheimer's. Phenolic acids and other flavonoids in apples protect it against damage by bacteria, viruses and fungi. Eating apples helps reduce the risk of cancer.

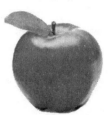

Apples. Yum!

Arginine

Arginine, also known as L-arginine, is an amino acid that is converted to spermine in the body with the help of manganese, Vitamin B-6, magnesium, and methionine. Low levels of spermine are associated with memory loss and senility, which can be averted by replenishing the body's supply of arginine. Turkey and chicken breast, soybeans, split peas, lentils, garbanzo beans, and cottage cheese are high in L-arginine.

Asparagus

Asparagus, consisting of long stalks, is known as the food of love by virtue of its distinctly phallic appearance. It has detox properties as it contains potassium, helps in maintaining water balance in the body. Asparagus is thought to treat some illnesses like asthenia, anemia, rheumatism, diabetes, and renal lithiasis, as well as being a natural aphrodisiac. Eating asparagus increases circulation in the genito-urinary system. It is rich in Vitamin E, a vitamin considered to stimulate production of sex hormones and may be essential for a healthy sex life.

Aspirin

Heart attacks caused by a blocked blood vessel in the heart and strokes caused by a blocked blood vessel in the brain are the most common causes of disability and death in the United States. Aspirin, known as the magical pill, has an immediate and lasting effect on blood platelets, making them less likely to clump together so that blood flows smoothly.

Astralugus

Astralugus tonic is believed to prolong life and boost libido. Practitioners of Chinese medicine use astragalus root to stimulate the immune system and the body's ability to resist and combat various diseases. It offers antioxidant benefits in people with severe forms of heart disease, relieving symptoms and improving heart function. Astragalus is believed to inhibit the spread and growth of cancer cells.

Avocado

People who keep low fat diet usually avoid avocado because it contains a lot of fat. But actually avocado is high in monounsaturated fat which reduces cholesterol level in the body. Avocado is a very good source of Vitamin E, which is essential for keeping your skin smooth and young looking. Avocado contains potassium which prevents high blood pressure. Avocado is great to use in sandwiches instead of butter spread.

> **I want to die young,**
> **at a ripe old age.**
>
> —Ashley Montagu

B

Ball

Throwing a ball up in the air and catching it as it comes down exercises sensory-guided movement activities, which hones the brains' visual, tactile and hand-eye coordination responses, with widespread positive impact on the brain. Playing ball with your kid or dog exercises and rejuvenates your brain.

Banana

In the traditional medicine of India and ancient Persia the golden banana is regarded as nature's secret of perpetual youth, promoting healthy digestion and creating a feeling of youthfulness. Bananas help retain of calcium, phosphorus and nitrogen—all of which regenerates tissues. Bananas contains invert sugar, which aids youthful growth and metabolism.

Bananas can be used as a dietary food for intestinal disorders because of its soft texture and blandness. Being bland, smooth, easily digestible and slightly laxative. ripe banana are highly beneficial in the treatment of ulcerative colitis, They relieve acute symptoms and promote the healing process. They are a treatment for constipation due to their richness in pectin, which is water-absorbent and bulk-producing ability. Bananas change the bacteria in the intestines to the beneficial acidophilus bacilli.

Bananas are beneficial in the treatment of anemia because of their high iron content. They stimulate the production of hemoglobin in the blood. Bananas are valuable in kidney disorders because of their low protein and salt content and high carbohydrate content. Juice from banana stems is a folk remedy for urinary disorders. It improves the functional efficiency of kidney and liver thereby alleviating the discomforts and diseased condition in them. It clears the excretion organs in the abdominal region of toxins and helps to eliminate them in the form of urine.

Basil

Holy basil can protect against the harmful effects of aging, according to research presented at a British Pharmaceutical Conference. Native to India, its extract has long been used in the ancient system of Ayurvedic medicine practiced in India and other parts of Asia as a rejuvenation drug, to promote a youthful state of physical and mental health. Researchers found that holy basil extract is effective at actively searching for and eliminating harmful molecules and protecting against damage caused by some free radicals in key organs such as the heart, liver and brain.

> **Youth is happy because it has the ability to see beauty. Anyone who keeps the ability to see beauty never grows old.**
>
> —Franz Kafka

Beauty

Looking at beautiful things soothes the soul and improves peace of mind by relieving tension. Enjoying beauty improves outlook on life and inspires hope. Bring beautiful things into your home. Enjoy beauty.

Beets

Ancient peoples believed that the color of beets was indicative of their power. In folklore, beets were eaten to aid the blood. Beets are high in carbohydrates and low in fat. They contains phosphorus, sodium, magnesium, calcium, iron, and potassium, as well as fiber, vitamins A and C, niacin, and biotin. Beet juice contains betaine, which stimulates the function of liver cells and protects the liver and bile ducts.

Red Beet is unique for its high levels of anti-carcinogens and its very high carotenoid content. They are an excellent source of folic acid and are loaded with antioxidants that helps the body fight against heart disease, certain cancers. Eating beets normalizing blood pressure, keeps the elasticity of arteries. The iron content of red beets, though not high, is of the finest quality, which makes it a powerful cleanser and builder of blood.

Bentonite Clay

Natural clay, especially the form known as "bentonite clay", has been used medicinally for hundreds of years by indigenous cultures. Primitive tribes have traditionally used various types of clay for removing toxicity. Animals in the wild have been observed licking clay as part of their everyday diet as well as rolling in it to get relief from injuries. Alternative medicine practitioners have used it as a simple but effective internal cleanser, especially of the bowels. Taken internally, liquid bentonite supports the intestinal system in the elimination of toxins. Clay is inert and passes through the body undigested.

Bentonite clay can take effect right away by binding to irritants in the gastrointestinal tract. It's a good idea to mix the clay with a cup of applesauce, which makes the clay more palatable and adds pectin—another binding agent.

Berries

Berries are packed with beneficial antioxidative compounds like vitamins C, E, beta-carotene and other nutrients that help curtail damage from cell-injuring free radicals circulating throughout the system. Berries contain memory-boosting nutrients. Blueberries contain proanthocyanidins that gravitate toward the striatum and boost spatial memory. Raspberries, strawberries and blueberries contain ellagitannins, which are found in the hippocampus, the brain's memory control center.

Beta-Carotene

Beta-carotene is an antioxidant and precursor to Vitamin A that prevents cancer, strokes and heart attacks by helping to keep arteries clear. It stimulates immune functioning that destroys tumors and prevents cataracts. Beta-carotene destroys singlet oxygen, a powerful free radical that damages cell structure. It is found in carrots, sweet potatoes, apricots, and spinach.

Biking

Since so many people are out of shape low impact exercises like biking are highly recommended for people who live sedentary or nearly sedentary lives as a way to get started on the path to fitness.

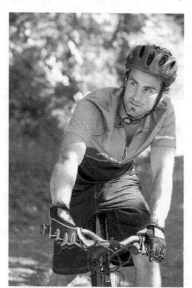

Biking is a great workout for the entire body, especially the lower body. Regular biking can significantly decrease your risk for heart disease. Health experts suggest that you should do aerobic exercise at least three times a week, keeping your heart rate elevated for at least twenty minutes at a time.

Because biking is a low-impact activity it doesn't cause a lot of stress on joints, making it a good exercise for people who may have limited range of motion or may not be able to handle an exercise like running, which puts a lot of stress on the joints. Biking can also reduce cholesterol and can help lower blood pressure, which is a major health concern for millions of people. Biking is therapeutic for the mind and spirit. It is fun and can increase your happiness quotient.

Biking is a great workout.

Bioidentical Hormone Replacement Therapy

Bioidentical hormone replacement therapy (BHRT) is the treatment of the hormone deficiencies caused by menopause with the use of molecules identical to the endogenous female hormones. The primary bioidentical female hormones are estradiol and progesterone.

Reduced production of estradiol in menopausal women is associated with hot flashes, vaginal dryness, poor memory, insomnia, and depression. Estrogen replacement can relieve these symptoms and slow or partially reverse medical disorders that are associated with the loss of estradiol including osteoporosis, atherosclerosis, vaginal atrophy, dementia, and depression. However, the Women's Health Initiative study showed an increase in breast cancer, heart attacks and stroke in women given conventional hormone replacement therapy. BHRT advocates argue that progesterone, unlike many progestins, may protect women not only from uterine cancer, but also from breast cancer.

Blueberries

Researchers at Tufts University rank blueberries number one in antioxidant activity when compared to 40 common fresh fruits and vegetables. Blueberries contain many plant compounds that combine to make this sweet fruit an antioxidant superstar. Their antioxidant, anti-aging, and anti-inflammatory effects protect you from premature aging. Blueberries keep us looking young, provide us with dietary fiber, and help protect us from cancer, eye problems, and age-related diseases. And it has only eighty calories a cup.

Blueberries have been shown to have a positive effect on slowing aging. In animal studies, blueberries appear to reverse some aspects of brain aging. The antioxidant and anti-inflammatory properties of blueberries build a protective coat around the brain to fight signs of aging and deterioration. There is also evidence that blueberries may help to prevent Alzheimer's disease and other neurological disorders.

Anti-inflammatory properties of blueberries appear to prevent and relieve arthritic symptoms, while the nutrients in blueberries strengthen blood vessels, leading to healthier blood pressure levels and heart health. The manganese in blueberries supports strong bones and its Vitamin C supports the immune system. All these factors contribute to the anti-aging capability of this amazing fruit–the blueberry!

Blue-Green Algae

Blue-Green Algae is touted as a super food because it is one of the most nutritional natural foods available. It is organic, easily digested and full of antioxidants. Algae is a kind of bacteria that lives in the water and manufactures its own food through photo-synthesis and is rich in minerals and has a higher concentration of beta-carotene than broccoli. Blue-green algae contains about sixty percent vegetable protein, and provides all the essential amino acids. It is a rich source of calcium, iron, Vitamin B-12, enzymes and antioxidants, making it an ideal food for both adults and children—even pets.

Blue-green algae has anti-aging effects because it has high concentration of antioxidants and can combat more free radicals and toxins. It is an energy booster with has rejuvenating effects. Greater concentration and focus—increase in energy and clarity of mind

Algae helps digestion by coating the stomach lining and is packed with digestive enzymes. Because it is a complete food, there are less cravings, which aids in weight loss. Its detoxifying features help us to sleep better. Regular consumption of blue-green algae improves memory. Eating blue-green algae helps us to stay fit and feel young and vigorous.

Boating

A survey found boaters expressed a greater degree of satisfaction in several key areas of life than their non-boating counterparts. Boaters said that they have greater satisfaction with their physical fitness and overall health, as well as the physical fitness and health of their children. Taking the helm and assuming the role of captain fosters leadership qualities and gives us a feeling of being in command. Spending time on the water brings peace and relaxation reducing stress. Life is better with a boat.

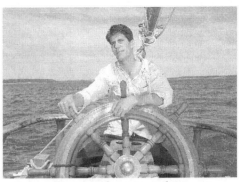

Boating is restorative.

Brahmi

The Sanskrit name *brahmi* is loosely translated in *The Yoga of Herbs* by Ayurvedic experts David Frawley and Vasant Lad as that which "gives knowledge of Brahman, or Supreme Reality." This herb promotes mental calm and clarity while improving memory and concentration. According to Frawley and Lad, "brahmi helps awaken the crown chakra and balance the right and left hemispheres of the brain." A satisfying tea is made by adding a half teaspoon of brahmi powder to a cup of hot water, then add honey to taste.

Brain Diet

Eating lean protein, low glycemic carbs, vegetables, especially leafy vegetables, and drinking generous amounts of water is good for your brain. Foods high in omega 3 fatty acids, such as fish—especially salmon and tuna, avocado, walnuts, blueberries, broccoli, green tea, oatmeal, which balances blood sugar, red bell pepper, spinach, and turkey are all good for keeping your brain youthful.

Brainwave Synchronization

The brain is a muscle that can be trained like any other muscle. You can make yourself smarter, more mentally alert, and increase your brain's performance by subjecting it to the right stimuli. Scientists have identified a "frequency following" response in which the human brain has a tendency to change its dominant EEG frequency towards the frequency of a dominant external stimulus. Such a stimulus might be a pulsing sound such as a beating drum, or a pulsing light like a strobe.

Brainwave entrainment synchronizes brainwaves with the frequencies in sound waves, which the brain follows and emulates. The theory is that by manipulating the frequencies you hear, the brain is pushed to operate at peak performance. Specially-crafted sounds influence brainwaves, resulting in sharper thinking, more energy, greater relaxation, and better problem solving skills. A google search of brainwave entrainment, as it is called, will take you to many brainwave training programs.

Breakfast

Breakfast is the most important meal of the day. Consuming a good, hearty breakfast helps the body get ready for a day of activity. The first meal acts to "jump start" and to keep metabolism working at a higher rate throughout the day. Blood sugar levels rise and remain higher longer after a hearty breakfast.

The higher caloric intake at the breakfast meal allows the body to function better all day, and the impact of a good breakfast helps the body become less hungry at later meals. Calories burn faster in the morning, following the breakfast meal, and the body metabolism slows down near bedtime.

Youth extending benefits of eating breakfast include a boost in concentration, energy and productivity levels. Eating high fiber breakfast foods like cereal, fruit, grains, nuts, and yogurt give you needed bulk in your diet, last longer, help you feel full and less hungry longer. High protein breakfast foods like eggs, milk, and meats are good breakfast foods. Eating breakfast improves overall nutrition, and helps reduce the risk of heart disease and regulate cholesterol.

Breathe

Breathing slowly and deeply relaxes the body and releases tension and anxiety. Breathing brings in oxygen, especially to the brain, which boosts mental clarity. Deeply exhaling helps to flush out CO_2 and other toxins. Mentally focusing on the breath is a way of expanding consciousness beyond the ego, promoting a transcendence experience.

Brewer's Yeast

Brewer's yeast is one of the few complete foods—though it doesn't taste that great. It is an excellent supplement to the diet. Brewer's yeast is almost pre-digested and is similar in this regard to other phyto-foods, like spirulina, chlorella, green barley extract and blue-green algae.

Brewer's yeast is low in fat, sodium, calories, and carbohydrates. It is a natural source of Vitamin B complex and highly concentrated amounts of protein, as well as being loaded with other healthy vitamins and minerals. It is high in folic acid, potassium, thiamin, niacin, chromium. Consumption of brewers' yeast reduces stress, promotes better metabolism and lowers cholesterol.

Adding a tablespoon to fruit juice is the simplest way to add brewers' yeast to your daily diet. It can also be added to meat loaf, salads, casseroles, cereal, and soup. Add the yeast at the end of the cooking process to prevent the Vitamin B complex from being destroyed. When first using brewer's yeast, start slow, with only a teaspoon full at first because it can cause lots of gas in the beginning. As you adjust to the taste, work your way up to larger quantities.

Brown Rice

People who eat brown rice tend to be leaner and have a lower risk of heart disease than those who don't. Brown rice is packed with antioxidants, phytoestrogens, and phytosterols that help prevent coronary disease. Brown rice provides the body with needed vitamins, minerals, fiber, and carbohydrates, which is the body's main fuel.

Buddhism

Buddhism focuses on the balanced interaction between the mind and the body, which is believed to be a prerequisite for healthy longevity, whereas disease results from imbalance and disharmony. The Buddhist approach to health and wellness is its emphasis on spiritual strength of the mind to overcome illness and disease. Buddha believed that you heal yourself through a drastic change in lifestyle and healthy attitudes towards the real meaning of life and existence.

Age is opportunity no less,
Than youth itself, though in another dress,
And as the evening twilight fades away,
The sky is filled with stars, invisible by day.
—Henry Wadsworth Longfellow

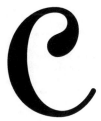

Cabergoline

Cabergoline enhances dopamine levels—a feel-good hormone—
while decreasing prolactin levels—a peptide hormone that regulates lactation and orgasms. It is believed that after ejaculation a
man's prolactin level rises. Recent studies indicate that cabergoline
can increase libido, orgasm and ejaculation for men. Wow!

Calcium

Calcium is a mineral that keeps bones from becoming brittle,
lowers blood pressure, protects the heart, and inhibits cancer.
Calcium prevents saturated fat absorption, which lowers LDL
cholesterol and reduces cancer cell proliferation. Studies have shown
that aging is associated with calcium imbalances, which leads to
osteoporosis, a debilitating disease associated with the elderly.

A Dutch study revealed a new mechanism where the hormone klotho, found in cerebrospinal fluid, urine and blood, helps
control blood calcium concentrations by regulating the amount
of calcium that is allowed to enter cells. Activation of the calcium
channel by klotho may form the link between the negative calcium balance observed in the elderly. Animal studies have found
that when klotho is removed, the animals undergo premature

aging. Calcium rich foods are very important to any anti-aging diet plan. Natural sources of calcium include cheese, yogurt, milk, kale, broccoli, and tofu.

Caloric Restriction

Caloric Restriction (CR) is a diet in which calorie intake is reduced without any reduction in nutrition. When you eat fewer calories, you slim down. Being overweight, or carrying excess body fat is harmful to long term health and increases risk factors for diabetes, cancer, and Alzheimer's. If you are overweight, you will have a shorter, less healthy life. CR has been proven to extend life span up to forty percent in rodents and primates. CR lowers risk for most degenerative conditions of aging. Particularly beneficial late in life CR reduces inflammation and muscle loss, cleans cells and reduces DNA damage, protects the heart against aging, and slows immune system aging and the progression of Alzheimer's disease.

A well-planned calorie restriction diet reduces intake of calories by twenty to forty percent, while still obtaining all the necessary nutrients and vitamins. Mild CR may be as easy as adopting a much healthier diet, taking a few supplements and not eating snacks. A helpful tactic for those practicing calorie restriction is to drink a glass of water when first feeling hungry. If you are still hungry twenty minutes later, then maybe it's time to think about eating. Half the time, you were just thirsty, however.

Cannabis

Cannabis is a euphorigenic plant. Eu in "euphoria" is the Greek word for "well," as in wellness. Euphoria engendered by cannabis blends relaxation, lightheartedness, optimism, and a sense of safety. Mental stresses, worries, and concerns recede into the background, giving way to feelings of insight, wonder, and pleasure in social contact, delight in simple things, and attention to the enjoyments available here and now.

The most notable aspect of the cannabis "high" is enhancement of the senses. Colors, and the contrasts and complementaries between them, become brighter and more vivid. Sounds acquire greater depth, texture, and dimension, and the spatial and harmonic relations between them become more pronounced, leading to absorbed fascination with music. The psychoactivity of cannabis promotes a keener awareness of bodily states, physical sensations, and physiological processes that are normally ignored. It can increase the pleasure derived from stretching, exercise, or yoga, from the relaxation and comfort felt in moments of repose, and can even infuse with joy an act as simple as breathing.

Cannabis' psychoactivity engenders a detached, distanced point of view that allows a person to observe emotions, thought processes, sensations, and desires with a sense of neutral objectivity. In this state of letting go it is easier to disentangle oneself from the unrelenting obsession, compulsive cogitation, and shortsighted viewpoint that characterize our usual attachment to issues of concern. Fluidity of mental processes and optimistic viewpoint can help people form new perspectives on things. The cannabis high is well-known for promoting humor and laughter. Humor heals the mind by refreshing perspective and keeping our viewpoint balanced; it heals the body by inspiring laughter.

Carnitine

Carnitine, also known as l-carnitine, acetylcarnitine, is an amino acid compound produced naturally in the body. L-carnitine promotes the burning of fat in the body, thus sparing proteins and carbohydrates from being used as muscular fuels.

Carnosine

Carnosine is a multifunctional dipeptide made up of a chemical combination of the amino acids beta-alanine and L-histidine. Long-lived cells such as neurons and myocytes—muscle cells—contain high levels of carnosine. Muscle levels of carnosine are correlated with maximum life spans. Carnosine levels decline with age. Muscle levels decline sixty-three percent from age ten to age seventy, accounting for the normal age-related decline in muscle mass and function. Since carnosine acts as a pH buffer, it protects

muscle cell membranes from oxidation under the acidic conditions of muscular exertion.

Carnosine enhances the calcium response in heart myocytes,
which enables the heart muscle to contract more efficiently. Aging causes irreversible damage to the body's proteins through a
mechanism is called glycation. Glycation is an underlying cause of
age-related decline, including neurological, vascular, eye disorders
and unsightly wrinkled skin.

Carrot Juice

Carrot juice has a lot of anti-aging benefits. It is a powerful antioxidant. It is high in beta-carotene, which converts to Vitamin-A
in the body and is very good for the eyes and skin. It's high content of Vitamins C, B, E, D and K, proteins, potassium, calcium,
phosphorus, zinc, aluminum, sodium, manganese, iron, copper
and other minerals gives carrots very good anti-inflammatory,
anti-cancerous and anti-aging properties.

Centrophenoxine

Centrophenoxine, also known as Lucidril, is a nootropic or "smart
drug". Its two active ingredients are DMAE and p-chlorophen-
oxyacetate, which work together to reduce lipofuscin or cellular
debris in the neurons of the brain and central nervous system. It
enhances the brain's ability to use glucose and accelerates information processing by facilitating nerve transmission across synapses.
Centrophenoxine breaks down into DMAE—an antioxidant—in
the blood stream, which also increases production of acetylcholine—a neurotransmitter.

Change Your Mind

Age often brings rigid thinking. Values and preferences deter-
mined in youth have continued unexamined for decades. What
we think determines who we are and how we feel. Youth is fluid
and changeable; old age is rigid and fixed. Change your mind and
your reality changes.

Take an opinion or preference you've had for a long time that is somewhat mundane to practice on. Then purposefully change your mind about it. Perhaps you have always disliked cooked carrots, for example. Work up an argument as to what's good about cooked carrots. Imagine how they taste—in a good way. Purposefully change your opinion of cooked carrots.

> **You are only as old as the last time you changed your mind. Change your mind often.**
>
> —Timothy Leary

Thinking in new ways prompts your brain to develop new neural pathways. A brain that is creating new pathways is a learning brain—a youthful brain. That old adage "use it or lose it" applies to your brain. When you stop using parts of your brain, neural pathways unhook and disappear. An unused brain is an old brain.

Cherries

Cherries are little anti-inflammatory pills. They contain Cox 2—inflammation and pain—inhibitors similar to those found in pain medications. Cherries also contain polyphenols, which keep platelets in the blood from clumping together. So cherries offer much of the benefits of pain medications without the risk of heart attacks and strokes associated with many pharmecutical drugs.

Chicken Soup

Chicken contains an amino acid called cysteine, which is released when you make the soup. Cysteine thins mucus in the lungs, aiding in the healing process. Chicken soup helps break up congestion and eases the flow of nasal secretions. Many say it also inhibits white blood cells that trigger the inflammatory response, which causes sore throats and the production of phlegm.

Chlorella

Chlorella is a natural whole food, with anti-aging properties. It is the highest food source of chlorophyll, which is a cleansing agent, and energizes the body with antioxidants, multivitamins and minerals. The unique fiber of chlorella binds to environmental toxins and heavy metals allowing them to be safely removed from the body.

The brain is the highest center of RNA concentration of the body, which declines with aging. When our RNA and DNA are in good repair and able to function most efficiently, our bodies are able to use nutrients more effectively, get rid of toxins and avoid disease. Cells are able to repair themselves and the energy level and vitality of the whole body is raised. Eating foods high in nucleic acids provides the material for the repair and production of human nucleic acids, and it is the breakdown of DNA and RNA in the cells that is believed to be one of the main factors in aging and degenerative diseases. Chlorella has the highest RNA, DNA, and chlorophyll content of any food.

Chocolate

Whenever Harry Potter or his friends are injured they are given chocolate to heal quickly. Research suggests that cocoa flavanols, which are more predominant in dark chocolate than milky versions, may lower inflammation, keep blood pressure in check, prevent platelets from clotting—which could prevent strokes and heart attacks—and boost brain power. Cocoa can improve blood vessel function, boosting circulation throughout the body and blood flow to the brain. The beneficial compounds found in cocoa may even reduce the formation of damaging clots, which may cause heart attacks and strokes. Eating chocolate may lower your blood pressure and cholesterol while providing an energy boost.

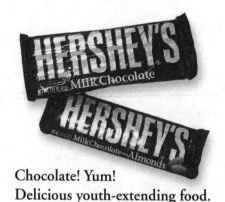

Chocolate! Yum!
Delicious youth-extending food.

Eating chocolate activates the systems in your brain that pump dopamine—the "feel-good" brain chemical. These systems enable learning and memory, and help keep your brain sharp and fit. Dark chocolate is a wonderful food that contains a large amount of antioxidants that protect your body from aging. Find good quality dark chocolate, learn to appreciate it, and have a bit of it each day.

Choline

Choline is a chemical similar to the B-vitamins, and serves various functions in the structure of cell membranes, protecting our livers from accumulating fat, and as the precursor molecule for the neurotransmitter acetylcholine. Choline improves mental performance and memory. Choline reacts with acetate to form acetylcholine, which is a neurotransmitter. Sources of choline include beef liver, whole egg, cauliflower, navy beans, tofu, almonds, and peanut butter.

Chondroitin Sulphate

Chondroitin sulphate is a substance that makes up the connective tissue in skin, tendons, ligaments, cartilidge. It has anti-inflammatory properties. As we age, our joints become inflamed, the cartilidge thins and we hobble about. Youth, by contrast, is nimble and quick. When we move easily without stiffness or pain, we feel and look youthful. Chondroitin sulphate enhances the synthesis of hyaluronic acid and cartilage production, thereby improving the quality of joint tissue. It inhibits enzymes that become overactive in joint degeneration and skin aging, destroying cartilage and connective tissue.

Chromium

Chromium, commonly sold as chromium picolinate, is a mineral that keeps blood sugar and insulin levels in check, which helps prevent heart disease and adult-onset diabetes. In turn, this regulates cholesterol levels and boosts immune system. Chromium bolsters insulin's ability to process sugar, thus normalizing levels of

both. It lowers detrimental LDL and raises beneficial HDL cholesterol, as well as stimulating T-cell and DHEA production.

Cinnamon

Cinnamon an excellent antioxidant that boosts brain power.
Just smelling the sweet odor of cinnamon boosts brain activity!
Research revealed that smelling cinnamon improved participants'
scores on tasks related to attentional processes, virtual recognition
memory, working memory, and visual-motor speed while working
on a computer-based program. There's indication that cinnamon
can enhance cognition in the elderly.

Cinnamon has anti-clotting ability. The cinnamaldehyde in
cinnamon helps prevent unwanted clumping of blood platelets.
Cinnamon's ability to lower the release of arachidonic acid from
cell membranes also puts it in the category of an anti-inflammatory food that can be helpful in lessening inflammation. Cinnamon
slows the rate at which the stomach empties after meals, reducing
the rise in blood sugar after eating. An Agricultural Research Service study showed that less than half a teaspoon per day of cinnamon reduces blood sugar levels in persons with type-2 diabetes.

Climbing

Stretching is vital for rock climbing. Good flexibility is essential.
Rock climbing improves body composition, flexibility, endurance and muscular strength. Stretching to reach the holds using
both finger and toes to get the grip and stay on the wall forces
the body to develop the necessary balance, improving hand-leg
co-ordination. Climbers quickly develop arm, back, finger, and
core strength as a result of the many reaches and holds that are repeated over and over through the completion of one climb. Rock
gyms are springing up in office parks across the USA, making it a
convenient way to meet up with friends after work without having
to travel a great distance.

Coenzyme Q10

Coenzyme Q10, also known as CoQ10, ubiquinone, ubiqui-nol-10, or vitamin Q, is a non-vitamin antioxidant nutrient that can be obtained in the diet or produced in the body. It helps in prevention of atherosclerosis, angina and heart attack. It protects cell membranes against free radicals, in conjunction with Vitamins E and C. It also seems to reduce clogging of the cardiovascular system. Coenzyme Q10 is an essential component of healthy mitochondrial function. It is incorporated into cells' mitochondria throughout the body where it facilitates and regulates the oxidation of fats and sugars into energy. It also protects tissues from damage due to oxygen deprivation. About ninety-five percent of cellular energy is produced in the mitochondria, which are the cells "energy powerhouses". A growing body of scientific research links a deficiency of CoQ10 to age-related mitochondrial disorders.

Coenzyme Q10 is produced in the body but production declines with age. Aging humans have been found to have over fifty percent less compared to that of young adults. This finding makes CoQ10 one of the most important nutrients for people over 30 to supplement. It is available in soy and olive oil, beef, peanuts, and fish

Coffee

Caffeine in coffee is one of the strongest legal stimulants available. Most people report improved mental alertness after drinking coffee. Caffeine stimulates production in the brain of the neurotransmitter norepinephrine.

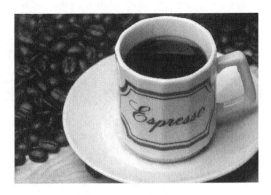

Coffee jolts alertness.

Studies show that coffee drinkers have a significantly lower risk of developing dementia than non-coffee drinkers. Some researchers believe it may lessen the risk of developing Parkinson's disease.

Cohabitate

People with close and loving relationships live healthier and longer lives. Studies from around the world show that loneliness is a major threat to health and long life. Virtually every gerontologist agrees that we can extend life significantly by creating a compatible and stable marriage with accompanying family life, and by cultivating many friends and being active in a number of social organizations. Cohabitate. Get roommates.

Collagen

Collagen is the main protein of connective tissue. Fibrous in nature, it connects and supports other bodily tissues, such as skin, bone, tendons, muscles, and cartilage. It also supports the internal organs and is even present in teeth. Collagen as the glue that holds the body together. Collagen works with elastin in supporting the body's tissues, to give form and provides firmness and strength. Elastin gives body tissues flexibility.

Collagen works with keratin to provide the skin with strength, flexibility, and resilience. As people age, however, collagen degradation occurs, leading to wrinkles and stiffness. As such, collagen is an important substance for fighting the visible effects of aging on the skin.

Competition

Kids and young people love to compete and do so naturally without hostility or angst. Competing is fun and fosters excellence and character development. Oldsters tend to avoid competition, preferring to plod along habitually, at their own pace. Competing just for the pleasure of stretching oneself is associated with youth. When competing we feel more youthful and more willing to take performance risks—to push ourselves.

Competition also has physical benefits. Researchers looked at the impact of training on the ventral and dorsal prefrontal cortex, which are the areas of the brain known to be associated with executive control—scheduling, planning, juggling multiple tasks and working memory. These areas are tied to cognitive declines in aging. Competition—pitting one's performance against others'— was central to the training. The study compared activation in the prefrontal cortexes of younger and older with younger adults, before and after training. After training they found less age-related differences. Older adults begin to look more like the younger adults in brain activation.

Complex Carbohydrates

Unlike simple carbohydrates that give your brain a "sugar high"—and may make you feel lethargic and mentally "fuzzy"— complex carbohydrates digest more slowly and provide a steady supply of energy to your brain, so that you feel sharper. Complex carbohydrates are found in foods like whole grain breads, brown rice, oatmeal, potatoes, and sweet potatoes.

Concentrate

Concentration is focused attention—the ability to direct attention to one single thought or subject, to the exclusion of everything else. When the mind is focused, energies are not dissipated on irrelevant activities or thoughts. Concentration has many uses and benefits. It assists in studying and understanding faster, improves the memory, and helps in focusing on any task, job, activity or goal, and achieving it more easily and efficiently.

Scientists have shown that the neurotransmitter acetylcholine, which is crucial to focus and memory, falls off with memory loss and is almost absent in Alzheimer's patients. Concentrating reinvigorates the controlled release of acetylcholine in the brain.

Ability to concentrate must be trained and exercised. Try this concentration exercise. Find a bench in a park or café where you can sit comfortably, undisturbed. Look straight ahead without

moving your eyes for about 60 seconds. Concentrate on everything you see, including in your peripheral vision. After about
60 seconds, blink your eyes to relieve any tension. Then, without
looking back, write a list of everything you remember seeing.
Then repeat the looking exercise and notice what you missed this
first time. Add these items to your list.

Curry

Turmeric, the yellow spice found in many curries, contains
curcumin, which has powerful anti-inflammatory and antioxidant
properties. Curcumin prevents the spread of amyloid protein
plaques in the brain and reduces accompanying brain inflammation. Amyloid plaque, along with tangles of nerve fibers, contribute to the degradation of the wiring in brain cells, eventually
leading to symptoms of dementia and Alzheimer's disease. Studies
indicate that consumption of turmeric or curry boosts cognitive
performance. Indian communities that regularly eat curcumin
have a surprisingly low incidence of Alzheimer's disease. Eating
curry two to three times a week may help prevent the onset of
Alzheimer's disease and dementia.

Cyronics

Cryonics is the science of using ultra-cold temperature to stop
issues from decomposing and preserve bodies with the intent of
restoring them to life and curing the disease that caused death when
technology becomes available to do so. It is expected that future
medicine will include mature nanotechnology, and the ability to
heal at the cellular and molecular levels. Cryonics involves stabilizing the viable brain of a patient who is legally deceased based on
cardiac death.

> **I want to be all used
> up when I die.**
> —George Bernard Shaw

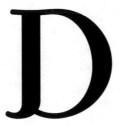

Dance

Dancing helps prevent dementia—both Alzheimer's disease and vascular dementia—according to the Einstein Aging Study. They compared reading, writing for pleasure, doing puzzles, board games or playing cards, group discussions, playing music, and dance and found that dance was the only physical activity that benefited the brain.

Dancing brings the benefits of exercising by burning fat and getting the blood flowing. However, the major benefits of dancing, according to the study, were attributed to the cerebral aspect of dance. Those who danced frequently—three or four times a week—showed seventy-six percent less incidence of dementia than those who danced only once a week or not at all.

Dancing is social and helps build bonds. It is relaxing and joyful, which makes us feel young, and sexy. Dancers get into the "zone", a kind of focused meditative state that rejuvenates the brain. Dancing with a partner usually involves physical touch, which trigger release of feel-good neurotransmitters. So dance your ass off every time you get a chance!

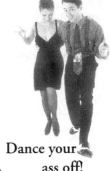

Dance your ass off!

Debauchery

Debauchery is immoral self-indulgence and engaging in extreme indulgence in sensuality. Often debauchery involves drunkenness. Being drunk helps to numb us to the sin of debauching—especially when women are involved. Boys will be boys.

Deer Antler Velvet

Deer Antler Velvet is prized in Chinese medicine as a sexual stimulant. It is the strongest of the 'yang' or 'male energy' tonics. Yang energy is an important aspect of sexuality and libido in both men and women, as well as a primary indicator of overall health, strength and vitality. Deer Antler is high in IGF-1 (insulin growth factor), which is linked to anti-aging factors in humans, including enhanced physical activity, muscle function, and testosterone and DHEA levels.

Deer antlers regenerate yearly and undergo extremely active mitotic growth. One hypothesis of deer antler's sexual enhancing effects, is that these quickly regenerating cells may act in a similar manner to stem cells, and provide young and rejuvenating cellular substance to the body.

Damiana

Damiana is an herbal medicine used by the ancient Aztec and Mayan civilizations. The extract binds to progesterone receptors, which may account for its use as a sexual enhancer. It is acclaimed to increase the frequency of intercourse, aid performance and heighten orgasm. Turnera aphrodisiaca is the species taken as a sexual stimulant for both sexes. Damiana is used for menstrual difficulties including headache, acne, insufficient flow, delayed menstruation in adolescent girls, irritability and lack of sexual desire It also helps to overcome sexual dysfunction, in addition to aiding the digestive system and toning the mucous membranes of reproductive organs. Jamaican folklore has it that when male goats eat damiana, their libido increases dramatically!

Daydream

A daydream is a visionary fantasy experienced while awake, especially one of happy, pleasant thoughts, hopes or ambitions. While we tend to think of daydreams as lazy, there are numerous examples of people in creative

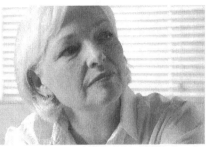

Let your mind wander.

careers, such as composers, novelists and filmmakers, developing new ideas through daydreaming.

Letting the mind wander can actually let the parts of the brain associated with problem-solving become active, a new study finds. MRIs of daydreamers show that the brain is quite active during daydreaming. Daydreaming seems to be an important cognitive state where we may unconsciously turn our attention from immediate tasks to sort through important problems in our lives.

Deprenyl

Deprenyl, also known as Eldepryl, Jumex, and selegiline, is a pharmaceutical that stimulates antioxidant activity and reduces the degradation of neurotransmitters, including dopamine and norepenephrine. It reduces fat-like deposits in the brain, called lipofuscin, that slow brain activity. Deprenyl is an established treatment for Parkinson disease and being researched as treatment for Alzheimer's disease.

Deprenyl extends maximum lifespan in animals and is a cognition-enhancer in normal, healthy animals. It is an antidepressant and acts as an aphrodisiac in male animals. Deprenyl is a popular anti-aging drug because it corrects so many of the typical problems associated with aging. It has been shown to help Alzheimer's disease patients live longer, and that can be attributed to its benefits to the brains of the patients. As the ultimate regulator of hormones and the immune system, the brain can exert its effect on every cell in the body. A youthful brain may be the key to a youthful body.

Desmopressin

Desmopressin, formerly known as vasopressin, is a peptide hormone found naturally in the brain and is partly responsible for the formation of memories. It is a peptide that is believed to deposit memories into the hippocanpus as they are learned.

Used as a nasal spray it is fast-acting to improve imprinting and short-term memory. Spraying 1 or 2 "puffs" of vasopressin into each nostril 15 minutes before recall or concentration is required markedly improves recall and the effect can then last for a few hours.

Destress

Stress wears out bodies and minds. Prolonged stress accelerates aging, making us look older than our age. Stress promotes cardiovascular ailments like high blood pressure, high sugar level and high cholesterol. The better that you manage stress the more fit, energetic and youthful you will feel. Do things that make you happy. Listen to music. Talk to friends. Breathe deeply. Relax your muscles. Take a warm bath. Take a warm bath with a friend, which is even more fun.

You can destress any time in any place by taking a deep breath. Here's how: Exhale strongly through the mouth, making a whoosh sound. Breathe in quietly through the nose for a count of four. Hold your breath for a count of six; then exhale with the whoosh sound for a count of eight. Repeat the cycle three more times. When standing in line, waiting on hold, driving in traffic, destress by taking a deep breath.

DHEA

DHEA, or dehydroepiandrosterone, is a natural sterone produced by the adrenal gland and similar in structure to androstenedione, testosterone, and estrogen. It is the most common sterone in human blood.

DHEA levels decline rapidly with age. Highest in the early twenties, DHEA begins to decline at around age 25. By age, 70 DHEA production nearly depleted. DHEA is thought my many to be the best over-the-counter anti-aging drug because it improves the metabolism of fat, decreases insulin resistance, increases lean muscle, and increases the efficiency of the immune system.

There is no cure for the common birthday.

—John Glenn

Alzheimer patients have low DHEA levels. Clinical trials have shown that DHEA helps brain neurons establish contact. DHEA seems to modulate cortisol level. Cortisol is a hormone that increases with age, induces stress and may affect many bodily functions, including damaging insulin resistance and the endocrine system including the hypothalamus. Maintaining healthy levels of DHEA to lower cortisol levels may be its most important role for aging and stressed individuals.

DIM

Diindolylmethane (DIM) is a phytochemical found in cruciferous vegetables including broccoli, cauliflower, cabbage and Brussels sprouts. Studies show that diets high in DIM balance the hormones estrogen and testosterone. It contributes significantly to the prevention of abnormal cell growth. Research has shown that DIM shrinks abnormal cells and tumors in areas of the body affected by hormone imbalance, like the breasts and prostate. It is generally considered better to get DIM from eating cruciferous vegetables than from supplements, which may be difficult for the body to absorb.

DMAE

DMAE—Dimethlylaminoethano—is naturally produced by the brain. DMAE can cross the blood brain barrier to enhance brain activity. Life extension advocates claim that DMAE increases life span and reduces DNA damage. It is an antioxidant. DMAE improves cardiovascular health, increases ability of the immune system, and seems to increase attention span. In one study, after 6 weeks of DMAE supplementation, students showed improved concentration at lectures and during examinations. Learning, memory, creativity, and verbal fluency are improved when taking DMAE

DMAE improves mood, reduces apathy and depression, improves memory and increases energy. DMAE is often added to skin-care products because it removes lipofuscin that causes age spots. DMAE is found in seafood such as anchovies and sardines, which may be why fish is often called "brain food".

**Youth is the best time to be rich,
and the best time to be poor.**
—Euripides

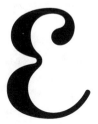

Enthusiasm

Youth is characterized by vigor and enthusiasm. When we express enthusiasm we look young and alive. Enthusiasm is excitement, passion, bouncing with energy. It signifies a whole-hearted devotion to an ideal, cause, study or pursuit. Enthusiasm is being visibly excited about what you are doing. Enthusiastic people are adventurous, constantly busy with many activities. Enthusiasm is magnet—its energy attracts others.

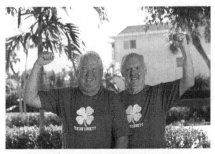

Enthusiasm rejuvenates.

The enthusiastic embrace life for its varied joys and wonders to live in the moment. Enthusiasm lifts us from fatigue to energy. Enthusiasm is characterized by a glowing face and sparkling eyes. The prime characteristic of enthusiastic people is radiation of positive energy. The smile of enthusiastic people lights up the room, heads turn and people gather around them.

Estrogen and Progesterone

Estrogen and progesterone are naturally occurring steroid hormones that play important roles in maintaining bone density and strength, sexual function, mental function. Research shows estrogen to help age-associated memory problems. Estrogen and progesterone are available in natural or synthetic forms, for oral or topical application. There is growing interest in plant-derived phytoestrogens, which have weak—but safe—estrogenic activity as a possible replacement for drug forms of estrogen.

Express & Emote

The young do everything with passion—emotion. Get in touch with your feelings and *feel!* To feel is to be alive, to experience. The next step is to express those feelings—including anger. Expressing anger constructively has been found to be healthy for the heart, whereas suppressing it is related to heart disease, especially among men. Nutrition and fitness specialist, Dr. Gary Null in a presentation at an anti-aging conference said "the mind-body relationship can't be healthy unless you're happy." Jump. Sing. Lament. Write poetry. Experience, express—enjoy life.

Exercise

Regular exercise keeps you slim and fit. Staying slim is one of the key factors to look young. Exercising tones your muscles and keeps them from sagging too early. Exercising burns extra flab and prevents bone loss. It helps to fight high blood pressure, cholesterol and promotes good sleep. Exercise increases cardiovascular capability. It keeps you slim, fit, stress free, while slowing aging. Exercising stimulates the brain to release serotonin, the "feel-good" neurotransmitter. Get on your bicycle, go to the swimming pool, take your dog for a walk, put a peppy tune on and dance your ass off.

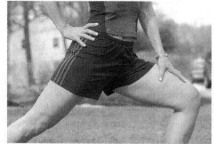

Exercise is the fountain of youth.

Exercise Your Brain

Exercise has positive benefits for the hippocampus, a brain structure important for learning and memory. When you work your brain it makes new connections; whereas when learning stops the brain disconnects synapses. Brain activities must be new and different for you to stretch your brain muscles. If you do a lot of crossword puzzles, doing more does not push the brain to create new connections. Instead play a video game. Take up ballroom dancing where you will learn new steps or play table tennis, which involves eyes, hands, feet, and thinking to all work together. Exercising the brain improves cognitive ability so that you can think better and remember more easily. Aerobic exercise, like dancing, increases oxygen loaded blood to flow to brain and feeds it. Exercise your brain for 15 or more minutes daily.

It was one of the deadliest and heaviest feelings of my life to feel that I was no longer a boy. From that moment I began to grow old in my own esteem and in my esteem age is not estimable.

—Anatole France

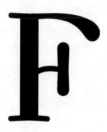

Face Lift

A face lift, or rhytidectomy, is a surgical procedure used to reduce facial wrinkles, eliminate telltale signs of aging, and improve the overall appearance of the face and jaw area. Patients whose skin is still relatively supple, and who are in good overall health, achieve the best results. With a laser face lift, there is no cutting, scarring, or anesthesia. Using laser technology, doctors resurface and tighten the outer layers of the skin, leaving patients with fewer fine lines and wrinkles. When you look younger, you feel younger.

Fake It Til You Make It

"Fake it till you make it" means to imitate the mood or behavior you want to establish. Curiously, pretending you are what you want to be helps you become it. Instead of getting trapped in a self-fulfilling prophecy of being old—which undercuts confidence—pretend you are already the person you want to be, which sets off a positive feedback loop. "Fake it till you make it" is often recommended as a therapy technique for combating depression.

Feel-Good Activities

When you feel good you feel young and vital. Bring more feel-good activities into your life. Make a list of activities that feel good when you do them. Notice what makes you feel good inside. When you feel a twinge of happiness, jot it down. Review the list and eliminate those things that are a little iffy in the feel-good department. Hone your list down to a collection of the good things in your life—things that bring you joy and provide fuel to keep going. Post your feel-good list on the frig where you'll see it often and make sure to engage in at least one or two feel-good activities each day.

Fenugreek

Diosgenin in fenugreek is an important precursor for the synthesis of a number of sex hormones, and exhibits estrogenic effects. The aromatic compounds in the fenugreek seeds have a maple syrup-like odor, which freshens the breath—an added advantage in sexual encounters. Harem women used fenugreek to increase the size and roundness of their breasts. The rich combination of nutrients in fenugreek include the steroidal saponin diosgenin, choline, trimethylamine—a sex hormone in frogs, Vitamins A, B-2, B-6, B-12, D, and essential oils

Fish Oil

Omega 3 improves memory, recall, reasoning and focus. When you eat foods high in omega 3 you'll feel like you're getting younger and smarter. Youth is characterized by smooth skin and baby-face-looks. Skin is actually the largest organ of the human body. One of the best ways to combat the formation of wrinkles and loss of collagen is to take in fish oil. Omega 3 and Omega 6 fatty acids play a critical role in promoting healthy skin.

Scientists have also found that fish oil containing EPA can limit the damage to the skin produced by overexposure to the sun and help to reduce the negative effect of UV rays. They help to regulate cellular function

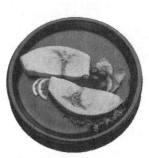

Eat fish for memory.

and maintain elasticity and suppleness in the skin. The American Heart Association recommends eating fish twice weekly, especially the fatty kind—salmon, herring, anchovies, mackerel and Tuna—which are rich in omega-3 fatty acids.

> To get back to my youth I would do anything in the world, except take exercise, get up early, or be respectable.
>
> —Oscar Wilde

Fish oil protects healthy blood flow in arteries. Omega 3 fatty acids, particularly EPA, have a positive effect on the inflammatory response, which prevents and relieves painful conditions like arthritis, prostatitis, and cystitis. Omega 3 fatty acids help to lower cholesterol, tryglicerides, LDLs and blood pressure, while at the same time increasing good HDL cholesterol, which adds years to your life expectancy. When plaque builds up on arterial walls and then breaks loose, it causes what's known as a thrombosis, which is a fancy way of saying clot. If a clot gets stuck in the brain, it causes a stroke and when it plugs an artery, it causes a heart attack. Omega 3 fatty acids break up clots before they can cause any damage.

Flavanols

Flavanols are phytochemicals found in cocoa, fruits and vegetables and have been shown to improve brain function and improve cognitive health. MRI studies have demonstrated that flavanol consumption improves blood and oxygen flow to the brain. Harvard researchers see hope for a treatment for dementia. Good sources of flavanols include citrus fruits, grapes, dark chocolate, red wine, blueberries, and green tea.

A nice cup of the right kind of cocoa holds the promise of promoting brain function as people age. Flavanols are often removed from cocoa drink mixes because they are bitter. The candy company Mars plans to market a line of products under the name CocoaVia®, which is high in flavanols. Other major chocolate companies, including Hershey's, are promoting the flavanol content of their dark chocolates. Flavanol-rich chocolate is a widely used in Hogworts.

Flexible Thinking

Youth questions just about everything. As time goes by we develop opinions, which come to feel so familiar and comfortable that we forget that they are opinions. They evolve into "facts" that we stop questioning.

Adapting requires flexibility. Flexible thinking is needed to deal with novelty but as we age we encounter less and less novelty. Things change less, we stop questioning our opinions, our thinking becomes more fixed. Flexible thinking must be cultivated.

Creativity expert Edward DeBono identified six styles of thinking: objective, emotive, supportive, possibility, critical and strategic. Each style has a corresponding question that taps the underlying thinking style.

Thinking Style	Question
Objective thinking	What are the facts?
Emotive thinking	What am I feeling?
Supportive thinking	What's working?
Possibility thinking	What's possible?
Critical thinking	What could go wrong?
Strategic thinking	What's the next step?

In "rut" thinking, we tend to go straight to critical thinking—What's wrong?—and to get stuck there. To other people this comes across as being closed and rigid, which we associate with aging.

Practice flexible thinking. You might write the six questions on a file card that you can post on the wall or carry in your wallet, that you can review when thinking about an issue or problem. One-by-one ask the questions to engage flexible thinking. Go through the process slowly, allowing your mind to mull over each question fully, while maintaining the style of thinking you are practicing.

Flirt

Flirting is adult play according to Barbara Bellman, author of *Flirting After Fifty*. It is a state of mind that includes confidence and playfulness. Flirting adds spice and panache to your life. Enjoy flirting—you

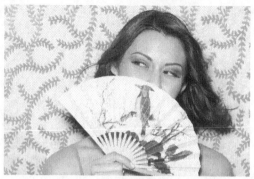

Go ahead—flirt! You'll feel great!

will feel young and sexy. All you have to do is to strike up a casual conversation with someone you find interesting. Bellman advises being playfully. It's just an opening to get a conversation going, not a commitment for life. Make the conversation about the other person rather than about you—and the more interesting you will be. Give your undivided attention, even if it's only for the moment. Everyone likes the feeling of being the center of the focus. Smile. People are drawn to people who look like they are welcoming and not rejecting. Make eye contact. Eye contact says you are fully present in the conversation.

As examples of flirting, Bellman suggests that you can give a compliment, like, "You have a beautiful smile". Make an astute observation, like, "I noticed you seem to be fascinated with that painting." "Ask for help, like, "I'm new to this neighborhood and don't know where…." Or self-disclose something, like, "I never know what to say at mixers like these, have you figured out the secret?"

Flow

An enjoyable altered state of consciousness known as the "flow state" can ensue when you are engaged in self-controlled, goal-related, meaningful actions. Musicians lose themselves in their music, painters become "one" with the process of painting. With complete absorption in an activity comes a suspension of time where we feel in control but not "controlling". This is flow, an experience that is at once demanding and rewarding—an experience that Mihaly Csikszentmihalyi demonstrates in *Flow: The Psychology of Optimal Experience,* is one of the most enjoyable and productive experiences we can have.

Flowers

Research shows that flowers are a natural and healthful moderator of mood. Flowers have an immediate impact on happiness. People receiving flowers experience delight and gratitude. Looking at flowers relieves depressed, and soothes anxiety. Flowers promote enjoyment and satisfaction. Bring flowers into your home and enjoy their beauty.

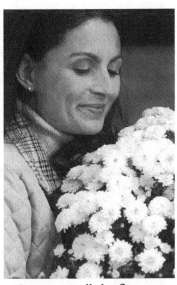

Stop to smell the flowers.

Problem-solving skills, idea generation and creative performance are facilitated in environments filled with flowers and plants. Other research revealed that flowers and plants in the workplace promotes productivity and problem solving. Flowers seem to refresh recent memory. Seniors performed higher on everyday memory tasks and experienced enriched personal memories in the presence of flowers. A Harvard Medical School study revealed that people feel more compassionate toward others, have less worry and anxiety, and feel less depressed when fresh cut flowers are present in the home.

Folic Acid

Folic acid is a B vitamin needed to make healthy new cells. Adequate folic acid levels are essential for brain function. Folate helps keep blood healthy. Not getting enough can cause a type of anemia, which is having fewer healthy red blood cells than normal. This makes it hard for your blood to carry enough oxygen throughout your body. Oxygen in the brain is essential for optimal cognitive functioning. Adding folic acid to the diet can help reduce age-related decline in cognitive function. High levels of folic acid are found in spinach, oranges, asparagus, and black-eyed peas.

Forgive and Make Amends

Forgiveness is releasing hurts and failures, guilt, shame, humiliation, anger and loss—letting it go. Forgiveness enables us to overcome anger and resentment and to let go of desires to punish or get even with those who have hurt us.

Research shows a correlation between thinking about hurtful memories and measures of the stress response—EMG, heart rate, blood pressure. The stress response diminished when subjects were encouraged to think forgiving thoughts. Research shows that forgiveness decreases anxiety, depression and grief. It decreases anger and negative thoughts. Forgiveness decreases heart rates, blood pressure and tension and is correlated with reduced chronic pain, cardiovascular problems, and violent behavior. With forgiveness comes increase in frequency of joyful experiences and hope. When you resume a connection with someone from whom you have been estranged you will be surprised at how liberated you will feel. Practice forgiveness.

Fo-Ti Root

Fo-Ti or "he shou wu" contains two anti-tumor agents, emodin and rhein. It is a tonic to the liver and kidneys and is said to maintain youthfulness and general good health. It strengthens the muscles and bones and keeps the hair color from premature graying. It is very beneficial for the nerves and is used for backaches, knee joint pain, traumatic bruises, and neurasthenia. Fo-Ti is a tonic for the endocrine glands, it improves health, stamina and resistance to disease.

Fruit and Vegetables

Fruits and vegetables are powerhouses of antioxidants. The body requires energy and raw material to maintain the cell's proper functions. Each cell needs the proper food to keep it strong. Cells die and replace themselves at various intervals. When a cell hasn't had the

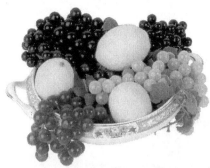

Powerhouse of nutrition.

right nutrition it will replace itself with a weaker cell, called degeneration. When a cell has an abundance of energy and the right raw materials the cell will replace itself with a stronger and better cell, called regeneration or anti-aging. Fruits highest in antioxidants include cherries, red grapes, oranges, plums, raspberries, strawberries, blackberries, blueberries, raisins, and prunes.

Youth is a circumstance you can't do anything about. The trick is to grow up without getting old.

—Steve Keyser

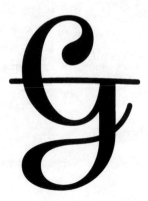

Games

Playing games keeps cognitive skills healthy. Solving puzzles, including trivia games, crossword puzzles, Sudoku, even charades enhance brainpower. Solving puzzles exercises the brain, stimulating it to make new nerve connections.

Playing physical games and sports is also a great way to keep both your body and mind healthy. Simple exercise routines maintain balance, flexibility, endurance and strength. Group games and sports also give the brain a workout, as you anticipate other people's actions and working together. Find games and activities that suit your level of physical ability and play often.

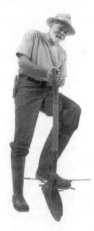

Gardening

Spending time in the garden is a rewarding hobby. Gardens are sensual places that engage all our senses, encouraging us to be more in touch with ourselves and in tune with nature's slower, gentler rhythms. Simply spending time in a garden, enjoying the sights, sounds and smells, can invoke a sense of belonging and spiritual peace. When we nurture a garden, we increase our connection and our sense of wellbeing. Remember to bend at the knees, get some ergonomic hand tools, avoid the midday sun and drink plenty of water. And take time to smell the roses.

Gardening is a pleasant, low impact workout. Weeding burns around 200 calories an hour. Planting burns 250 calories per hour, which is more than golfing without a cart. Hoeing and raking burn about 350, about the same as dancing. When digging, your metabolism really sours, burning 450 calories per hour, similar to taking a bike ride. Working in the garden can be a form of strength training and build endurance and flexibility.

Garlic

Garlic is an entire pharmacy made up of over 400 chemicals. It has strong anti-aging properties, is a powerful antibacterial and antiviral agent, is a potent blood thinner, and is full of antioxidants for good health.

Many believe that eating garlic blocks cancer and prevents its growth once started because it retards cellular decay and helps in retarding growth of abnormal cells. Garlic lowers cholesterol, fights against blood clots, boosts immune functions, and acts as an anticoagulant and antioxidant. Aging lowers immunity, which is why old people are more prone to catching infections and falling sick. The anti-bacterial and anti-viral properties of garlic thwart these agents from multiplying in the body to cause sickness. The beneficial anti-aging properties of garlic are at their strongest when the garlic is raw. If you don't like the sharp, bitter taste, swallow the cloves whole as you would vitamins.

Gerovital

Gerovital, sometimes called GH3, is the original anti-aging drug introduced in the 1950's by Romanian gerontologist Dr. Ana Aslan. The active agent in Gerovital is procaine, which is believed to have anti-aging properties by lowering brain levels of MAO (monoamine oxidase) activity. MAO is an enzyme in the brain that increases with age that degrades key neurotransmitters such as noradrenaline, dopamine and serotonin, causing them to decrease with age—with a concomitant loss of brain functions, e.g. memory, attention span, hormone regulation, as well as an increase in depression.

Early antidepressants were MAO inhibitors but had a potentially serious side effect called the "cheese effect," where eating certain foods (such as cheese) and drinks rich in tyramine while taking the prescription MAO inhibitor could lead to high blood pressure, even strokes. In contrast, Gerovital is a weak, reversible MAO inhibitor that does not exhibit the cheese effect. A Duke University study reported that most patients taking Gerovital felt a greater sense of well-being and relaxation, slept better, experience relief from depression and the discomforts of chronic inflammation disease. Other benefits reported in journals include stabilizing brain cells in ways that reverse normal aging-related membrane deterioration, increasing general intracellular metabolic rate, and increasing intracellular DNA levels. The effect of these actions is to clean and dilate blood vessels to improve circulation. Results are first seen in the hair and nails.

Ginkgo Biloba

Ginkgo is remarkably effective at protecting mitochondria from damage. Mitochondria generate most of the cell's supply of adenosine triphosphate (ATP) or cellular energy, and are involved in a range of other processes, such as signaling, cellular differentiation, cell death, as well as the control of the cell cycle and cell growth. Research has shown that as we age, mitochondria become less efficient at producing energy and more efficient at generating damaging free radicals. This vicious cycle is now believed to be a major contributor to the aging process and memory loss. Even more impressive, Ginkgo has been shown to preserve mitochondria structure and function in aging animals, as well as to also significantly extend their life span!

Ginkgo is one of the oldest living tree species and has been used for centuries in traditional Chinese medicine. Regular use of Ginkgo extract improves memory and slows down early Alzheimer's. It lowers blood pressure, raises beneficial HDL cholesterol, and improves blood circulation through arteries, veins and capillaries.

Ginger

Ginger oil, which has a warm, spicy-woodsy odor, has been used as a healing remedy for thousands of years. It is used to reduce muscular aches and pains, increase circulation, relieve bronchitis and whoop-

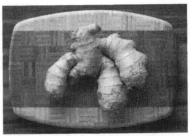

Ginger soothes inflammation.

ing cough, nervous exhaustion, and to stimulate appetite. Ginger has powerful anti-inflammatory properties. It is used to increase energy, appetite, and for anti-aging purposes.

Aging is accompanied by gradual lowering of immunity, making it easier for the bacteria and virus to attack the body with greater intensity. With an infection comes inflammation—the forerunner of many diseases. Inflammation means swelling, redness, pain and extreme discomfort. Ginger can put a stop to all these symptoms. Since ginger can control inflammation to a significant level, the cells suffer less from the consequences of free radical hits and the symptoms of aging are considerably delayed.

Ginseng

In ancient times, the miraculous ginseng root was reserved for emperors and kings who believed it to be a source of youth. Ginseng is reputed to reduce fatigue, stress, mental anguish and nervousness. It soothes the soul.

Ginseng's active complex of ingredients is ginsenosides, which control hormone activity and the regulating mechanism of nerves. They influence blood pressure and insulin production, and increase metabolism, which is probably the reason for improved cerebral activities, alertness and memory. Ginseng is thought to be a cure all herb and an aphrodisiac. When hormones are balanced properly people are healthier and have healthier sexual appetites. Combined with the increased energy that ginseng gives, it's common for ginseng to promote an increase in sexual activity for both men and women. It is often used to reverse impotency problems in men.

The best time to take Ginseng is in the morning, making it a good alternative to coffee because it increases stamina. Ginseng seems to be more potent if you drink a lot of water throughout the day. Exercise also seems to increase its potency. Ginseng makes an excellent "pick me up" for both physical and mental stamina when mixed with Cayenne and Gota-Kola.

Green Tea

Research has shown that drinking green tea is helpful in fighting cancer, arthritis, tooth decay and other chronic illness. Green tea is a strong antioxidant. It contains catechins, which fights viruses and slows aging. Epigallocatechin gallate (EGCG), an antioxidant found in green tea, is said to be 100 more times more effective than vitamin C and 25 times more effective than Vitamin E at protecting cells. Green tea extract helps maintain cellular DNA and membrane structural integrity. Research findings show that green tea inhibits the development of undesirable cell colonies. The active constituents in green tea are powerful antioxidants called polyphenols (catechins) and flavonols. One cup of green tea may provide 10-40 mg of polyphenols and has antioxidant effects that are greater than a serving of broccoli, spinach, carrots, or strawberries.

Glutathione

Glutathione (GSH) is a naturally occurring antioxidant and contains cysteine, which breaks down free radicals and prevents new ones from forming. It is important for intracellular health. Animal and laboratory studies have demonstrated that glutathione has the potential to fight almost any disease, particularly those associated with aging, since free radical damage is the cause of many of the diseases of old age. It rejuvenates, boosts immunity, blocks cell damage, prevents adult-onset diabetes, protects against air pollution, cigarette smoke, heavy metals, and alcohol. Glutathione is found in avocado, watermelon, asparagus, grapefruit, acorn squash, brussels sprouts, cabbage, cauliflower and broccoli.

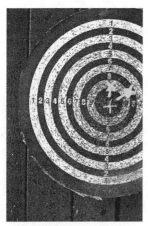

Target to shoot for.

Goals

Youth is forward looking, while old age looks backward. When seniors speak of things they would like to do, they often use their age as an excuse for doing nothing. "What? At my age!" "Oh. It's too late for that!" Striving for something generates enthusiasm and sense of empowerment—potency. The ability to effectively set goals throughout life is one of the most important skills that any of us can have. Goals help us to get moving and to keep moving. Goals add to the excitement of life.

A goal is a target to shoot at. It is a result toward which effort is directed. It is an outcome to be achieved. Goals focus your efforts because there is a target to shoot for. They tell you where to shoot and which way to go. Goals create momentum and get us moving.

> **A man is not old as long as he is seeking something.**
>
> —Jean Rostand

Set a goal and look at it every day. Break it into small steps. Take a small step and you are in motion. When you are moving towards something you value and want, you feel youthful and fully alive.

Go With The Flow

Going with the flow is rolling with the punches and accepting change without getting angry or frustrated. It's taking what life gives you, rather than trying to mold life into what you want it to be. Enjoy life as a flow of change, chaos and beauty. Accept change and imperfection. Accept things as they are. The world is constantly changing; we are a part of that change. See things as funny, rather than frustrating.

Gotu-kola

Gotu-kola is a plant found throughout Africa and the East and, like ginseng, is considered an adaptogen. Gotu-kola has been used to treat obesity, varicose veins, wounds, and some skin conditions. Taken with calamus root, it may improve memory and mental clarity. It may improve attention and concentration, have an anti-stress tranquilizing effect, stimulate the brain by increasing blood flow, detoxify the body, and energize the cells. Consequently, gotu-kola is said to increase longevity.

GPC

L-alpha-glyceryl-phosphoryl-choline (GPC) aids in the synthesis of several brain phospholipids, which increases the availability of acetylcholine in various brain tissues. GPC's brain-boosting qualities have been studied for their ability to enhance overall brain function. In young patients, for instance, it seems to improve memory and the ability to pay attention. GPC's most important role is in the production of choline, a water soluble B vitamin that is important for the brain and nervous system and has been shown in studies to help protect against cognitive decline typical in aging.

> Life is a series of natural and spon-
> taneous changes. Don't resist them—
> that only creates sorrow. Let reality
> be reality. Let things flow naturally
> forward in whatever way they like.
>
> —Lao-Tzu

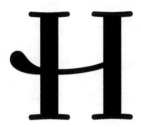

He-Shou-Wu

According to legend, an impotent 58 year old Chinese man was trapped by a flood in the mountains for seven days where he ate He-Shou-Wu. Amazed, he developed a strong sexual desire and subsequently fathered several offspring. He lived to 130 and died with black hair. A modern Chinese herbalist Li-Chung-Vun is claimed to have lived 256 years of age, was married 24 times and looked like a young man of 50 when he died. His secret was drinking He-Shou-Wu and ginseng daily.

He-Shou-Wu is widely used in Chinese herbal medicine as a tonic to prevent premature aging by tonifying kidney and liver functions. It brings up Jing—vital essence, nourishing the blood, and fortifying the muscles, tendons and bones. It strengthens and stabilizes the lower back and knees. He-Shou-Wu is widely used in Asia to maintain the youthful condition and color of the hair and is a popular tonic for enhancing sexual drive and fertility in both men and women. It increases sperm count and helps build more semen, even in old age it helps build ova in women.

He-Shou-Wu herbal tea can be prepared from the processed roots of the herb, by boiling about three to five grams of the herb in a cup of water for about 10 - 15 minutes. The decoction must then be strained.

HGH

Human growth hormone (HGH) is a protein produced by the pituitary gland that stimulates the body to grow and develop until the end of adolescence. HGH is the "master hormone" controlling many organs and body functions and is responsible for stimulating tissue repair, cell replacement, brain functions, and enzyme function. It is responsible for vitality, energy and the health benefits we associate with youth. It has a remarkable ability to reverse the effects of aging in humans. After adolescence HGH continues to be produced, primarily during sleep, to assist with tissue repair, healing, muscle growth, brain function, bone strength, energy, metabolism, and physical and mental health. However, its production falls off as we age.

HGH reduces body fat, for example. In a study overweight men who did not alter their personal habits of eating, smoking, or exercise, treated with HGH lost an average of 14% of their body fat, while gaining an average of 8.8% lean muscle mass. Their skin became firmer and they experienced a localized increase in bone density. The study concluded that HGH appeared to reverse the effects of aging by 10-20 years!!!

A synthetic HGH given by injection is exceedingly expensive, costing $12,000 to $225,000 annually, making HGH use for anti-aging is impractical. The body does not absorb HGH taken orally. However, oral ingestion of the amino acids arginine, histidine, glutamine, ornithine, methionine, phenylalanine, and lyisine may stimulate HGH production.

Higher Power

Research has shown that all forms of spiritual belief and faith exert a powerful benefit on health and long life. In a study of a thousand long-lived Americans, the Committee for an Extended Life-span found that almost without exception, every single longevous person has strong spiritual beliefs. The same study found that over fifty percent of all long-livers turn their problems over to a higher power relying on it to guide them toward the best possible solution. While their faith safeguards them from stress, they are able to relax and enjoy living.

Honey and Cinnamon

Honey is the only food on the planet that does not spoil or rot. Honey is always honey, although when left in a cool dark place for a long time it will crystallize. Never boil honey or put it in a microwave because the heat kills the enzymes in the honey.

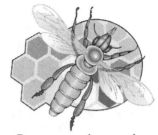

Boost your immunity.

As we age, arteries and veins lose their flexibility and get clogged; honey and cinnamon revitalize the arteries and veins. A mixture of honey and cinnamon can help. Make a paste of honey and cinnamon powder, apply on bread, instead of jelly and jam, and eat it regularly for breakfast to reduce the cholesterol in the arteries and possible heart attack.

Honey plus cinnamon taken regularly can cure arthritis. A Copenhagen University treated 200 patients with a mixture of one tablespoon honey and half teaspoon cinnamon powder before breakfast. 73 patients were totally relieved of pain, and most most of the others reporting considerable pain reduction.

Honey plus cinnamon reduces cholesterol and soothes the symptoms of the common cold. It also soothes upset stomach and boosts the immune system.

Tea made with honey and cinnamon powder, taken regularly, arrests the ravages of old age. It keeps the skin fresh and soft and increases life span. Senior citizens, who take honey and cinnamon powder in equal parts, are more alert and flexible.

Hope

Hope is a belief that positive outcomes and circumstances will manifest. It is the feeling that what is wanted can be had or that events will turn out for the best. Hope can be passive in the sense of a wish, or active as a plan or idea. Despair is the opposite of hope. Despair leads to depression, even death. Youth is characterized by hope—belief that wondrous things will come about, whereas old-age is often characterized by despair and just hanging on.

Hope comes from seeing there is something out there. Plans let you believe again. Prepare a list of things you want to do, give yourself something to look forward to, give yourself targets to get through each day and pat yourself on the back for your progress however modest it may be.

Horny Goat Weed

Horny Goat Weed is a time-tested aphrodisiac that increases libido in men and women, and improves erectile function in men. The leaves of the plant contain a variety of flavonoids, polysaccharides, sterols and an alkaloid called magnaflorine. And while the exact way that horny goat weed works remains unknown, the plant has long been employed to restore sexual fire, boost erectile function, allay fatigue and alleviate menopausal discomfort.

Animal studies indicate that horny goat weed may work by increasing nitric oxide levels, which relaxes smooth muscle and lets more blood flow to the penis or clitoris.

Hormone Replacement Therapy (HRT)

Hormones are chemicals produced from cholesterol, amino acids and proteins from endocrine glands that work as messengers between the brain and body organs. HRT adjusts the body to aging. It improves skin and body moisture, and increases sexual drive so you feel young and energetic.

HRT is most commonly used by women following menopause. Decreased levels of estrogen during menopause may cause hot flashes, vaginal dryness, sleep disturbances, or other bothersome side effects. HRT seems to help prevent osteoporosis, heart disease, short-term memory loss, depression and other diseases in post-menopausal women.

Hugging

Something so simple as a hug can
make you feel connected, supported
and loved. A hug can reduce heart
disease, cut down stress and promote
longevity. Hugs increase levels of
oxytocin, a "bonding" hormone, and
reduce blood pressure—which cuts the
risk of heart disease.

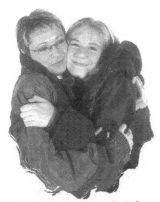

A University of North Carolina
study discovered that hugging has
measurable benefits for the heart. Researchers asked 38 couples to sit close

Hugging extends life.

to one another, talk, and then hug. Afterwards, women showed
somewhat lower levels of cortisol and lower blood pressure, while
both men and women had increased levels of oxytocin.

Oxytocin, also called the "cuddle hormone", is a chemical
associated with a range of health benefits, which shows a marked
increase in the blood supply after just ten minutes of warm,
supportive touching. It calms. Hugging triggers production of
the hormone, which, in turn, promotes a desire to touch and be
touched.

Hyaluronic Acid

Hyaluronic acid has been called the "key to the fountain of youth"
because it has been noted that at least some people who ingest
a lot of it in their diets tend to live to ripe old ages. Hyaluronic
acid is a component of connective tissue whose function is to
cushion and lubricate. In skin tissue, hyaluronic acid is a jelly-like
substance that fills the space between collagen and elastin fibers.
Facial lines and features can be corrected using hyaluronic acid
implantation, including frown lines that run between the eyebrows, marionette lines at the corner of the mouth, worry lines,
crow's feet, deep smile lines that run from side of the nose to corners of the mouth, and cheek depressions. Hyaluronic acid is also
known to decline in its availability with advancing age.

Hyaluronic acid implantation is temporary. After injection into the skin, hyaluronic acid gradually breaks down and is absorbed by the body. Augmentation usually lasts three to nine months, so that repeat treatments or "top-up" treatments are needed to maintain results. Most people have 2 to 3 treatments per year.

Hydergine

Hydergine is derived from *Claviceps purpurea,* a fungus that grows on rye. It prevents free-radical damage in the brain, increases the brain's blood supply, delivery of oxygen, and metabolism—all of which lead to improved memory. It is the first drug to show efficacy as a treatment for Alzheimer's disease and dementias.

Hydergine is touted as a "smart" drug for use in enhancing mental abilities and improving intelligence, but its mechanism of action is still not clear. Studies indicate that it has the ability to enhance memory and learning. It improves a range of cognitive abilities, such as concentration and recall, and helps to prevent damage to brain cells from insufficient oxygen. Hydergine mimics the effect of a substance found in the brain called nerve growth factor, which stimulates the growth of new dendrites. Many neuroscientists believe that intelligence is correlated with the number of interneural connections in the brain. Studies have demonstrated that hydergine actually increases cortical thickness in the brain and that it also raises levels of the neurotransmitter dopamine.

> **Youth is not a time of life, it is a state of mind. You are as old as your doubt, your fear, your despair. The way to keep young is to keep your faith young. Keep your self-confidence young. Keep your hope young.**
>
> —Luella F. Phean

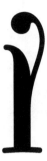

Immune System

The immune system is vital to maintaining health and youthfulness. It fights off disease carrying germs and bacteria that enter the body. Antibodies and antitoxins—the foot soldiers of immunity—recognize these foreign bodies and attack them using leukocytes—white blood cells.

When the immune system weakens, infections can take over, making you more susceptible to colds, viruses, and more serious illnesses. The immune system can only work at optimal capacity when it is properly cared for. To do this you must help accelerate immune system recovery, increase cellular health, strengthen and promote overall cellular integrity and reduce depletion of crucial nutrients. Vitamins, minerals, enzymes are essential for the functioning of the human immune system.

Israel researchers made discoveries that suggest rejuvenation of the immune system might slow or partially reverse the aging of the brain. These researchers believe immune system T-cells enter the brain to carry out functions beneficial to the brain. They have shown that immune cells carry away toxins and have evidence that immune T-cells stimulate brain stem cells to produce new nerve cells—neurogenesis. They have shown that the same immune cells may also be key players in the body's maintenance of the normal healthy brain. Their findings suggest that the immune system's T-cells—which recognize brain proteins—enable the "neurogenic" brain regions, like the hippocampus, to form new nerve cells, and maintaining your cognitive capacity—to keep you youthful!

Ice Skate

Ice skating is relaxing, therapeutic and improves concentration. Skating develops coordination, poise and good posture. Fitness benefits of ice skating include improved blood circulation, muscle tone, stamina and increased flexibility. It provides aerobic exercise equal to walking, running, swimming, bicycle riding, jogging—all of which build up the stamina of your body.

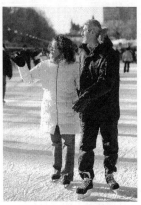

It's invigorating!

Ice skating is an inexpensive activity that provides an excellent source of exercise and entertainment. Ice skating develops grace while building confidence. With the first shaky hands-free ride around the ice, confidence is built. The ice will be conquered. You can skate at indoor rinks or out of doors. Skating out in crisp cold air is exhilarating from the muscular system to the respiratory system to the circulation system. The benefits to the mind—the rejuvenation of the mental state—is immeasurable.

Idealism

Idealism is characteristic of youth. It is the tendency to envision things in perfect but unrealistic form. Idealists have utopian views. They are romantic and starry-eyed filled with hope and optimism. Oldsters tend to be cynical with an attitude of jaded negativity, and a general distrust of the integrity or professed motives of other people. They show contempt and tend to be bitterly or sneeringly distrustful, contemptuous, or pessimistic. Cynical people deflate us, making us feel small and silly. Resist the pull of cynicism and purposefully cultivate idealism—yours and that of your fellows.

Imagination

Imagination it is the ability of the mind to build mental scenes, objects or events that do not exist, are not present or have happened in the past. Memory, itself, is actually a manifestation of imagination. Imagination helps provide meaning to experience and plays a key role in the learning process. It strengthens your creativity and improves your ability to plan, whether it be a family picnic or a corporate venture. Imagination helps to break out of rut thinking and mental boxes. It gives the ability to look at any situation from a different point of view, and enables us to mentally explore the past and the future.

You can travel anywhere with the speed of light without any obstacles in your imagination, freeing you even if only temporarily from tasks, difficulties and unpleasant circumstances. When imagining engage all of your five senses and your emotions for a powerful experience. Imaging provides mental stimulation that exercises the brain and keeps us youthful.

Impishness

Impishness is acting whimsically, mischievous and punkish. It is a playful naughtiness, possibly a bit annoying. Peter Pan and Huck Finn, both boys who refuse to grow up—to grow old—are delightfully devilish, impish rascals who do quite a bit of teasing of their friends and elders. Children, puppies and kittens are impish rascals who delight us, even while causing consternation.

> **Great is the man who has not lost his childlike heart.**
> —Mencius

Improvise

Improvising is to act without preparation, possibly suddenly, even hastily. It is extemporaneous, free-form, unpremeditated, spur-of-the-moment action. Improvisation often leads to new views and practices, to creative break-throughs. Improvisation can be applied to most artistic, scientific, physical, cognitive, academic activities. It breaks up rigid mind-sets. People who improvise are seen as youthful, creative and fun to be around.

Planning, of course, is good and needed, but can become a stifling straight-jacket. Practice improvisation whenever possible. Do
things on impulse, the spur of the moment. Ad lib. Play it by ear.
Take things as they come. Improving involves breaking out of old
habits and patterns and exercises your brain in new ways, which
prompts the brain to create new neural pathways, which grows the
brain. A growing brain is a youthful, smart brain. Lighten up and
make it up as you go along and you will be amazed at how young
you will feel in the doing.

Innocence

Innocence is a state of unknowing naivety, connoting an optimistic view of the world. It is wide-eyed wonder characteristic of
youth. As we make our way through life and the world it is easy to
become jaded—worn out, wearied and fatigued, dulled or satiated
by overindulgence, dissipated. Jaded is the sister of cynicism—
scornful negativity and distrust of others. Some think cynicism is
the mark of sophistication. But don't be fooled. Jaded cynicism is
a frequent characteristic of oldsters. It is closed and negative. The
open innocence of youth is vastly more appealing but all too hard
to retain. Cultivate innocence and you'll find that wonder and
mystery will return to you.

Innovate

Innovation involves introducing something new, making changes
in something established. Innovators are often viewed as pio-
neers—people out on the front lines, getting bugs in their teeth.
Innovation is new, fresh. It is the opposite of established, routine,
static, old, customary, usual, habitual, beaten path, ruts, treadmill
—all of which dull us. Innovation always involves risk because the
new approach may not work. Risk-taking is exciting, stimulating
and makes us feel more alive—more youthful.

Inspire

To inspire is to exert an animating, enlivening, or exalting influence. To inspire is to motivate, move, cause, stimulate, encourage, influence, persuade, spur, be responsible for, animate, rouse, instill, arouse, cause, produce, excite, prompt, induce, awaken, give rise to, ignite, kindle, enkindle, infuse, hearten, enliven, imbue, spark off, energize, galvanize, gee up, inspirit, fire or touch the imagination. It takes cleverness, genius, imagination, imaginativeness, ingenuity, inspiration, inventiveness, originality, resourcefulness, talent, and vision. To inspire is to breath life into ideas and into people. It lifts you and those you inspire. Inspire others and be open to inspiration and you will feel more alive and youthful.

Interest

Youth is characterized by being open and interested, whereas oldsters are too often closed and bored. When you show interest in others they feel special and generally like you back. You can show interest in others by smiling and making eye contact. Most important is to ask questions about the person, their activities, likes and dislikes.

Nothing is more flattering than having someone show interest in you. Showing interest is inviting and encourages others to approach you. Ask others questions and listen to the answers. People absolutely love to talk about themselves, and therein lies the key to being interesting. As you ask them questions about themselves, be on the lookout for any common interests that you may have with them, as this will open up an conversation that is of interest and a lot more relaxed and personal for both of you.

Talk to strangers. Strike up conversations with people you encounter during your day—someone on the subway, your waitress, car mechanic. Dare to be different. People are attracted to eccentric people. However, be careful to not be wacky or weird so that you spook folks.

Irreverence

Youth is questioning and typically disrespectful of authority—irreverent. Youth "talks back" and is impertinent. Youth is often cheeky, cocky, contemptuous, flippant, fresh, iconoclastic, impious, impudent, immature, insolent, mocking, out-of-line, punkish, rude, sacrilegious, sassy, and saucy. And why not? With age, we learn to be "PC", which is stifling. Take back your inner irreverence. Prance around. Talk back. Ask provocative questions. Laugh. Use taboo words. Step over the line. Push the envelope. Moon 'um. Flip 'um the bird. Stick out your tongue! Blaaaaaa!

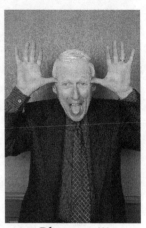

Blaaaaaaa!!!

Many of the most successful men I have known have never grown up. They have retained bubbling-over boyishness. They have relished wit, they have indulged in humor. They have not allowed "dignity" to depress them into moroseness. Youthfulness of spirit is the twin brother of optimism, and optimism is the stuff of which American business success is fashioned. Resist growing up!

—B. C. Forbes

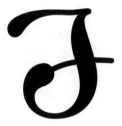

Jatamansi

Known as "the mental soother", Jatamansi can soothe an anxious, agitated mind. This Himalayan-native herb has similar calming properties to its relative, valerian, without the dulling effects. It's a powerful brain tonic and memory booster and a useful herb for palpitation, tension, headaches, restlessness, used for promoting awareness and strengthening the mind. Jatamansi is a useful hair tonic and is commonly used in hair oils, promoting hair growth and luster. It is also used in oils and pastes that improve complexion and general health of the skin. Jatamansi stops fermentation and gas in the intestines so you don't have to worry about polluting the environment with your methane gas emissions after eating a lot of beans and other musical fruit.

Jazz

Jazz is a style of music characterized by a strong but flexible rhythmic understructure with solo and ensemble improvisations on basic tunes and chord patterns and, more recently, a highly sophisticated harmonic idiom. Native to America, jazz was created mainly by African-Americans in the early 20th century through an amalgamation of elements drawn from European-American and tribal African music. It is characterized by the use of improvisation, bent pitches or 'blue notes', swing and polyrhythms.

During prohibition when the sale of alcoholic drinks was banned, illicit speakeasies became lively venues of the "Jazz Age", an era when popular music included current dance songs, novelty songs, and show tunes. Jazz got a reputation as being immoral and many members of the older generation saw it as threatening traditions and promoting the decadent values of the Roaring 20s.

Jazz is an experimental, exuberant music—youthful. To jazz someone is to give pleasure and excite, to exaggerate as is so often the case with youth. When things are jazzy they are more enlivened and exciting. Listen to jazz when ever you want to get your foot taping and your juices flowing.

Jitterbug

Jitterbug refers to a type of dance to Rock 'n' Roll, Bee Bop and Jazz. Also called "swing", it is an exuberant fast-paced dance characterized by rotations and switches, quick movements, with swinging arms and freewheeling acrobatic swings and lifts. Jitterbugging provides an incredible aerobatic workout that makes you feel high on life and half your age. Want a new lease on life? Take a stint at Camp Jitterbug. Learn the Lindy Hop dance camp. What could be more fun and invigorating?

Call of the Jitter Bug

First thing you must do is get a jug,
Put whiskey, wine and gin within,
And shake it all up and then begin.
Grab a cup and start to toss,
You are drinking jitter sauce!
Don't you worry, you just mug,
And then you'll be a jitter bug!

—Cab Calloway

Jigsaw Puzzles

Like every muscle in your body your brain needs to be exercised on a daily basis. Putting together jigsaw puzzles exercises the brain. Completing one requires fine visual judgments about where pieces belong. It entails mentally "rotating" the pieces, manipulating them in your hands, and shifting your attention from the small piece to the "big picture."

Jigsaw puzzles develop your abilities to reason, analyze, sequence, deduce, logical thought processes and problem solving skills. They also improve hand-eye co-ordination and develop a good working sense of spatial arrangements. The hunt for pieces forces your

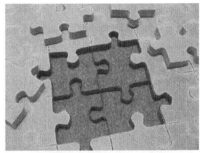

Puzzles exercise your brain.

brain to memorize what each piece looks like, or should look like, and to conceptualize what kinds of pieces you are searching for in order to complete the picture. Doing this repeatedly reinforces short-term memory. Studies have shown that individuals over the age of 70 who enjoyed puzzles as a hobby were 2.5 times less likely to develop Alzheimer's disease. And to top it off, jigsaw puzzles are fun!

Juice

Vegetable and fruit juices are fat-free, nutrient-dense beverages rich in vitamins, minerals and naturally occurring phytonutrients that promote good health. Phytonutrients are compounds in fruits, vegetables and other plants that have disease preventative and disease fighting properties. Juicing allows you to add a wider variety of vegetables in your diet. Drink vegetable juice for breakfast. Vegetable juice is superior to fruit juice due to the high sugar content of fruit. Vegetable juice doesn't raise insulin levels like fruit juice, except for carrot and beet juice, which function similarly to fruit juice.

Make your own juice. Celery, fennel, and cucumbers are the easiest to digest. As you get "into" juicing, add the more nutritionally green leafy vegetables. Vegetable juice does not have much protein or fat, so you might add an egg to the mix. Blend in ground seeds, like pumpkin and flax seeds, for increased satiety. Add algae, like chlorella or spirulina, which are packed with nutrients.

Two types of juicing machines are available. A juicer separates the juice from the plant pulp, which is discarded. However, the pulp contains considerable nutrients and beneficial fiber. An alternative is the Vita-Mix®, which pulverizes or juices the entire plant so that you drink the pulp, which is full of fiber that helps your intestines to function and clear out debris.

Jump Rope

Jumping rope is the best activity to help fight heart disease, obesity, type II diabetes, and osteoporosis while improving strength and fitness. In addition to the obvious physical benefits, jumping rope is fun. There are always new footwork patterns that you can develop and practice.

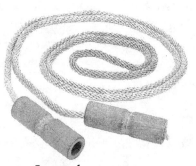

The jump rope is a tried and true method for improving conditioning and coordination. If you have never jumped rope before, expect a challenge. There can be some initial frustration. It is important that you become proficient with the rope before using it as a conditioning tool. View your rope sessions as

Jump the years away.

skill workouts. You need to develop skill with the rope, and then add it to your conditioning arsenal. Just try to skip for 20 seconds without tripping on the rope. Keep the intervals brief, and stop before becoming fatigued

Juvenescent

Juvenescence is being or becoming youthful. It is being young in appearance or having the power to make one young or youthful: a juvenescent elixir.

> **An inordinate passion for
> pleasure is the secret of
> remaining young.**
>
> —Oscar Wilde

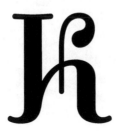

Kava Kava

Kava Kava, scientifically known as *Piper Methysticum*, and sometimes called the "intoxicating pepper" operates via neurotransmitters, which sends feel-good vibes to the brain. The kavalactones in Kava cause changes in brain activity similar to that of anti-anxiety drugs, but without the sedative or hyponotic effects. It aids muscle relaxation, increases concentration, decreases insomnia, lowers inhibitions.

Animal studies show that kava affects the limbic system, an ancient part of the brain and the principal seat of emotions. In other words, it may alter the way emotions are processed rather than having a tranquilizing, depressing action. It is often recommended for pain and stiffness, anxiety, insomnia, pain and jet lag. Traditionally chewed or crushed to form a liquid, Kava is now commonly found in capsules, teas and liquids aimed at reducing a variety of stress and anxiety related conditions and illnesses.

Kelp

Kelp or seaweed is a green marine plant has substances necessary for the immune system's functional integrity. It contains five vitamins: B-12, niacin, choline, carotene and alginic acid, plus 23 minerals, making it one of the most health-enriching supplements available. Often called a "miracle plant", kelp has many thera-peutic properties and is a good protective food, valuable in over-coming poor digestion, preventing and overcoming goiter, and rebuilding and maintaining the proper function of all glands.

Kelp can correct mineral deficiencies. A teaspoonful sprinkled on your food twice a day provides salt and vital trace minerals. Kelp is a good source of protein and a rich source of iodine and iron. Iodine is needed for proper functioning of thyroid and blood cell function aids in brain development, helps prevent osteoporo-sis, and increases metabolism.

Kissing

Kissing is great for self-esteem because when kissed we feel ap-preciated, which improves state of mind. Kissing slows the pace of aging. Medical studies have revealed that people who kiss their partner goodbye each morning live five years longer than those who don't. Kissing and touching releases endorphins, increases the levels the love hormone, oxytocin, which soothes anxiety and stress, and lowers the cortisol or 'stress' hormone, which has a claiming effect and produces a sense of well being.

Kissing burns two to three calories a minute and can double your metabolic rate. Research results have shown that three passion-ate kisses a day, lasting twenty seconds or more each, will cause you to loose a pound. Kissing exercises thirty facial muscles, helping to prevent baggy cheeks. It brings a glow to your face making you look more youthful.

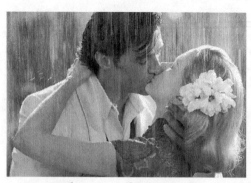

Kissing creates an adrenaline rush so that the heart pumps more blood. Research has shown that frequent kissing stabilizes cardio-vascular activity, and decreases blood pres-sure and cholesterol.

Pucker up to lower stress.

Kissing is good for the teeth, too. During a kiss, natural antibiotics are secreted in the saliva, which washes bacteria off your teeth, which breaks down plaque build-up.

Kiwifruit

Kiwifruit offers a rich nutritional reward in a small, delicious package. Inside of this small, brown, fuzzy egg-sized fruit you'll find semi-translucent green flesh and small black seeds around a white center.

Kiwifruit has a unique sweet flavor something like a combination of strawberries, pineapples and bananas. It has an unusually abundant amount of Vitamin C and other anti-aging antioxidants. Kiwifruit offers beauty benefits from stimulating collagen synthesis—vital to lovely skin—to maintaining healthy bones and teeth to protecting against wrinkles and premature aging. Because kiwis are antioxidant all-stars, they help neutralize free radicals, which otherwise do damage to cells that could lead to inflammation, cancer, and heart disease. On top of all of these benefits kiwi is a slimming fruit with only 92 calories in two medium fruit.

Knitting

Knitting, crochet, and other needle arts are traditional crafts dating back thousands of years. The rhythmic repetitive movements are soothing to help prevent and manage stress, pain and depression. Many argue that the repetitive movements of knitting activate the same areas in the brain as meditation and yoga, which have been shown to help prevent pain and depression. Pain specialists explain that the action of knitting actually changes brain chemistry, decreasing stress hormones and increasing feel-good serotonin and dopamine. Knit gloves, scarves, and sweaters, which you can give away and you'll probably get a bunch of kisses.

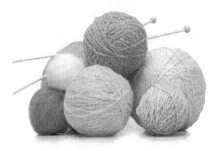

Knitting is soothing.

Kombucha

Kombucha is a fermented tea drunk for medicinal purposes. It is claimed to stimulate the immune system, prevent cancer, improve digestion and liver function and increase energy. Health claims for kombucha focus on a chemical called glucuronic acid, a compound that is used by the liver for detoxification. Although frequently referred to as a mushroom, which it resembles, Kombucha is not a mushroom; it's a colony of bacteria and yeast. Kombucha tea is made by adding the colony to sugar and black or green tea and allowing the mix to ferment. The resulting liquid contains vinegar, B vitamins and a number of other chemical compounds.

Care must be taken during preparation and storage to prevent contamination. Maintaining a correct pH is an important factor in a home-brew. Acidic conditions are favorable for the growth of the kombucha culture, and inhibit the growth of molds and bacteria.

The Food and Drug Administration cautions that the risk of contamination is high because Kombucha tea is often brewed in homes under non-sterile conditions. There are reports of adverse effects such as stomach upset and allergic reactions. Lead poisoning also may be a risk if ceramic pots are used for brewing—the acids in the tea may leach lead from the ceramic glaze.

Anyone who stops learning is old, whether at 20 or 80. Anyone who keeps learning stays young. The greatest thing in life is to keep your mind young.

—Henry Ford

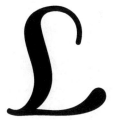

Laugh

Laugh long and laugh often. Laughing makes us feel happy, helping us to stay youthful. When we smile we stretch and exercise the muscles in our face. Laughing lightens our burdens, inspires hopes, connects us with others, and keeps us grounded, focused, and alert. Humor helps to keep a positive, optimistic outlook

Laughing relaxes the whole body. A good, hearty laugh relieves physical tension and stress, leaving your muscles relaxed for a long as forty-five minutes. Laughing decreases stress hormones and increases immune cells and infection-fighting antibodies, thus improving resistance to disease. Laughing triggers the release of endorphins, the natural feel-good chemicals. Endorphins promote an overall sense of well-being and temporarily relieves pain. Laughing protects the heart, by improving the function of blood vessels and increasing blood flow.

Create a list of three things that make you smile, every time you think of them. Items might

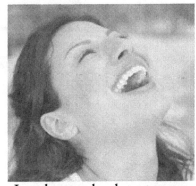

Laughter melts the years away.

Ha! Ha! Ha!
Ho! Ho! Ho!
And a couple of tra la las.
That's how we laugh
the day away.

—Munchkins
The Wizard of Oz

be scenes from a movie, a line from a book, a joke, an event. It doesn't matter where they come from, or what they are, so long as thinking of them makes you laugh. Then anytime you are mad, upset, sad, depressed, or just need a laugh, remember the things on your laugh list.

Laugh Exercise: Assume a comfortable sitting position on the edge of a straight back chair. Count to three and on "three", stand up quickly and laugh the biggest, deepest laugh that you can. Make sure to take a deep breath and to laugh so heartily that your teeth show. Sit back down and repeat the exercise several times. The fun of this exercise can be increased by doing it regularly with your family or coworkers at the office. Try this exercise with co-workers during a laugh break and see what happens!

Lasik and Lazer Vision Treatment

Eye disorders and diseases are common in older adults. Laser surgeries and other treatments exist to correct and even reverse some of these conditions. Cataracts, age related macular degeneration (AMD), diabetic retinopathy can be helped with lazer treatment.

Diminished vision, especially distance vision, usually begins in one's 40s. Before you know it you have your bifocals on a string around your neck, which makes you look and feel "elderly. If you leave home without your glasses, you squint and lean over to read price labels looking like Mr. McGoo in the grocery store—you feel like an old foggie! You look like one, too.

Standard lazer treatment for age-related near-sightedness is about a 10-15 minute painless procedure that transforms your life. No more glasses around the neck. No more squinting. Immediately you feel as if fifteen years dropped away. Wow! If you think that it is costly. Then consider this. Cleopatra, with all of her power and wealth could not buy—at any price—the new eyes that lazer treatment provides for a few thousand dollars.

Lean Protein

Eating protein prompts the brain to manufacture norepinephrine and dopamine—neurochemicals that promote brain alertness and keep you energized an feeling good. Good sources of lean protein include low fat milk and yogurt, hard cheeses, lean meats, and poultry.

Learning

Lifelong learning keeps us young by exercising and expanding our brainpower. When learning content different from our core knowledge base, the brain develops new neural pathways. The brain wires itself. The more you use your brain, the more wired it becomes. "Use it or lose it" is true for brainpower. When you don't use your brain enough, it begins to unwire itself. To stay youthful, challenge your brain with lifelong learning.

> **Learning is ever in the freshness of its youth, even for the old.**
>
> —Eschylus

Left Hand

Use your non-dominant hand when doing routine activities. If you're right-handed, brush your teeth using your left hand. Do this until it feels natural. Build your way up to more complex tasks, such as eating, tying shoes and so forth. Using your non-dominant hand to perform increasing complicated movements presses your brain to create new neural pathways as you establish control of your hand. A growing brain is a youthful brain.

Lecithin

Lecithin has an indispensable role in regulating the flow of nutrients and waste materials in and out of the cell. Lecithin is an emulsifying agent that enables fats and other lipids to be dispersed in water so it breaks down fats in the body. Lecithin is often added to candy, such as the malt nougat in the Mars Milky Way®, to keep it soft. Similarly, lecithin prevents the hardening of fats and bad cholesterol in the walls of the heart, the arteries and the veins, thereby promoting cardiovascular health. It also protects cell membranes from hardening. High concentrations of lecithin are found in the brain and prostate gland.

Lecithin improves brain function by providing acetylcholine, which is an important substance that helps brain cells continue to communicate effectively. Acetylcholine is found to be lacking in Alzheimer's patients. Increasing lecithin in the diet can help those suffering from Alzheimer's disease and boost memory.

The body only needs 30 to 50 grams of lecithin, which can be obtained by eating egg yokes, wheat germ, soybeans, fish, legumes, peanuts, whole grains and yeast. It is available as a supplement in capsules, as a powder or granules, which can be added to food. Taken in small doses, lecithin has no side-effects. However, if taken in high doses it can cause diarrhea, weight gain, headache, nausea, gastrointestinal problems, vomiting and dizziness.

Legumes

Legumes—beans, peas and lentils—are unsung heroes, packed with nutrients with very few calories. Legumes are a valuable part of a healthy diet, because they are low in fat, do not contain cholesterol, have a significant amount of fiber, and are high in protein. Legumes help regulate sugar, water and other aspects of metabolism. Sprouted legumes are an excellent source of vitamin C and

Legumes are unsung heros.

enzymes. A one-cup serving of dried peas or beans provides about one-fourth of an adult's daily protein needs. Always remember that beans are the musical fruit, the more you eat, the more you toot.

Lipoic Acid

Lipoic Acid is a highly potent antioxidant that counteracts reactive free radicals in the mitochondria, the power plant of cells where energy for all cellular activities is generated. Some scientists believe that mitochondrial free radicals play an important role in human aging, and have theorized that extra amounts of free-radical inhibiting compounds such as lipoic acid may help slow aging. Lipoic acid is also effective in recycling other antioxidants such as Vitamin E back into their original form after they detoxify free radicals. There is evidence that lipoic acid can reduce glycation damage due to excess glucose in the blood, which may be involved in aging.

Listen

Good listening skills help in understanding, thinking and remembering. When you focus your attention on what someone is saying, you release the neurotransmitter acetylcholine, a brain chemical that enables plasticity and vivifies memory. One technique for tuning up your listening is to set your television volume down a little from your normal volume. Concentrate on listening until you can follow the dialogue just as well as when the volume was higher. Then turn it down another notch to stretch your listening skills a bit further.

Live Like You Were Dying

Wake up! Life isn't forever. One day you will die. Live life here and now. It's easy to get caught up in the little annoyances and fuss over little things that don't matter. Tomorrow is not guaranteed, so live life today. Take advantage of the time you have here and make the best of it. Start doing things you have being thinking of doing. Do It Now!

Somebody should tell us, right at the start of our lives, that we are dying. Then we might live life to the limit, every minute of every day. Do it! I say. Whatever you want to do, do it now! There are only so many tomorrows.

– Pope Paul VI

Love

Happily married people live longer. Love promotes better heart health. In one study, despite high risk factors like high cholesterol, high blood pressure, and diabetes, men who felt loved by their wives experienced half the angina as men who felt their wives did not show them love. Feeling loved increases

> Learn to dial and tune your brain and you can enrich your sex life beyond your wildest dreams. The brain is the ultimate organ of pleasure.
>
> —Timothy Leary
> *Search for the*
> *True Aphrodisiac*

levels of the "anti-aging" hormone DHEA, which produces feelings of youth and vitality. Showing support and affection for loved ones seems to slow the aging process even more than receiving love does. Humans are wired for connection, and when we cultivate loving relationships, the rewards are immense: fewer colds and faster healing, less depression, lower blood pressure, less anxiety, and longer, happier life.

The brain is the primary sex organ. Falling in love stimulates the brain in the same way that cocaine does. Fall in love with your spouse again. Get giddy. Let yourself go. Find someone to fall in love with.

Lychii Fruit

Lychii fruit, also called Wolfberry, and Go-Qi-Zi, has traditionally been used in China for thousands of years for its rejuvenating effects on sexuality and fertility. Lychii is a small red berry which is dried and prepared as a tea. Scientific studies have found that polysaccharides found in Lychii fruit protect both male and female sex organs from free radical damage.

> A man's age is something impressive, it sums up his life: maturity reached slowly and against many obstacles, illnesses cured, griefs and despairs overcome, and unconscious risks taken; maturity formed through so many desires, hopes, regrets, forgotten things, loves. A man's age represents a fine cargo of experiences and memories.
>
> —Antoine de Saint-Exupéry

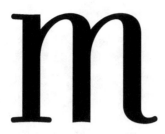

Maca

Organically grown maca root, also called *Lepidium meyenii*, is considered by top researchers to be a true adaptogen and touted as the "superfood of the Andes" by the natural products industry. Maca root helps rebuild weak immune systems, re-mineralize poorly nourished bodies, and increase energy and endurance.

Adaptogens raise the non-specific resistance in an organism and enable the body to enhance its power of resistance and adapt to external conditions. The legendary sex-enhancing radish-like root is employed into a Peruvian maca extract to increase strength, energy, stamina, libido and sexual function—a winning combination of health benefits.

Magnesium

Magnesium is a mineral that protects against free radicals, especially those that attack mitochondria, the energy-producing part of a cell. Magnesium lowers blood pressure and prevents heart attacks. It prevents diabetes and may even work to reverse it. Magnesium protects against coronary spasms, blood clots, and blood vessel constriction. It works with calcium and Vitamin D to keep bones strong.

Magnesium is found in whole grains, nuts, seeds, and legumes, or can be taken as a supplement. Most easily absorbed are magnesium chloride, aspartate, gluconate, or lactate. Men should consume just slightly more than women.

Make Out

Making out is kissing. Kiss your make out partner's face, cheek and neck. Hug. After a forehead or neck kiss is a great time to wrap your arms around your partner and give him or her a warm, affectionate embrace. Run your fingers through his hair along the scalp from front to back, all the way down to his neck. Smile and gently lean your forehead against hers and put your hand on her face. For an extra boost try making out at a drive in movie—assuming that you can find one. No? Then put a movie on your flat screen, throw a thick comforter and a few large pillows on the floor, get your partner and make out! Park benches and the back of buses are other good make out spots.

Make Over

Dress younger, sexier, slimmer, or just learn how to dress to flatter your figure. With a make over you can experiment with a new look and a new you. Wow! Give yourself a virtual makeover with celebrity hairstyles, makeup and accessories on one of the makever sites on line where you can use your photo and try versions looks: Try hairstyles, make up, and even clothing.

And make overs are not only for woman. Men, too, can undergo an amazing transformation with a new hairstyle or by cutting off that old, boring beard.

Meditate

Leading alternative medicine researchers have found that people who meditate achieve reduction in oxygen use, lower secretion of stress hormones, increase in immune factors, including blood leukocyte production, and calm brain wave activity. Other research has shown that regular meditation reduces anxiety and chronic pain, lower levels of cortisone, increase in cognitive function, lowered blood pressure, and reduction in the use of medical care and hospitalizations.

One study showed that people meditating five years were physiologically twelve years younger than their non-meditating counterparts in blood pressure, vision and hearing. Even the short-term participants were physiologically five years younger than the controls. The positive results endured in a follow-up study conducted ten years later.

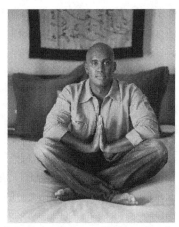

Meditate for youthful outlook.

How to Meditate: Go to a private, comfortable place by yourself where you won't be interrupted for 10-20 minutes. Sit down in a comfortable chair and close your eyes. Breathe deeply. Relax your muscles. Beginning with your feet and moving to your face, slowly flex and then relax your muscles. Adopt a calm, passive attitude, a neutral mind in which you don't judge yourself or others. Silently repeat a word or mantra to help stop your internal dialogue. When thoughts intrude, simply let them go and bring yourself back to your mantra. Sit quietly for a couple of minutes when you finish. Try to carry your calm, rejuvenating, meditative attitude into your daily activities.

Melatonin

Melatonin is a hormone that regulates daily life cycles. Some scientists believe that it is an "aging clock" that regulates senescence. Secreted by the pineal gland, located in the middle of the brain, in response to darkness, melatonin regulates daily and seasonal cycles of life. It is released every night as part of our time-dependent biorhythms to help induce sleep and recuperation from fatigue. While melatonin production declines with age, taking it in supplements may extend life span as well as youthfulness.

Melatonin is a highly potent antioxidant and considered by many to be a "miracle hormone" that pervades tissues throughout the body and boosts immune functions even in systems compromised by age, drugs and stress by stimulating production of T-cells in the thymus gland. It can ease insomnia, help overcome jet lag, protect tissues from damaging free radicals, help fight infections, reduce the rate of cancer, fight malignancies—and extend life.

Memory

Research into brain plasticity, which is the ability of the brain to change at any age, indicates that memory activities that engage all levels of brain operation—receiving, remembering and thinking—improve the function of the brain and slow rate of decline.

Exercising your brain can be fun. For example, go on a guided tour of a museum or another site of interest. Pay careful attention to what the guide says. When you get home, try to reconstruct the tour by writing an outline that includes everything you remember. Not only will you have a more memorable time, but in exercising your brain, you rejuvenate it.

A healthy mind is key in youth extension. Your brain is a muscle. It needs to be used and exercised. After reading an article in a newspaper, put it aside and do a self-quiz. Play memory games with your children or grandchildren, for instance. Enroll in brain fitness training, such as that sponsored by Posit Science, which offers a 40-hour scientifically developed program to improve memory and mental functioning.

Mid-Life Crisis

Mid-life crisis describes a period of dramatic self-doubt that is felt by some individuals in the "middle years" of life, as a result of sensing the passing of youth and the imminence of old age. Carl Jung believed that mid-life is key to individuation, a process of self-actualization and self-awareness and is a normal part of the maturing process. Spotting that first gray hair or noticing your pecks turning into flab can set off the crisis. "Oh my gawd, I'm getting old", you lament. This can set off the crisis—a time of transition when you to take stock of where you are in life and make some needed adjustments to the way you live your life.

You may experience a deep sense of remorse for goals not accomplished and a desire to achieve a feeling of youthfulness. Go with it and embrace your mid-life crisis. Yes, you've fallen into a rut. Break out and *live*. When you do you will surely feel ten years younger.

Move

When we live in the same place for a long time things begin to blend together and time shortens. We look back ten years and it seems like ten months. The longer we live there, the more time seems to compress. Yet, for the first several weeks and months after we move into a new home, time seems to expand. The first week seems almost like a month. So experientially, we get more time in life when we move often.

There is a lot of comfort in living in the same place for a long time. But comfort can lull us into a kind of chronic narcolepsy—walking sleep. One day you wake up like Rip Van Winkle to discover twenty-five years have passed and you hardly remember much of it.

Youth fills its days with stimulating activities. A year in your life when you were a college student seems much longer and fuller than a year in your life at fifty years old. You can regain some of that stimulating fullness by moving. Yes, moving is stressful and triggers a lot of emotion. When we feel emotions we feel more alive—younger. Moving is an opportunity to get rid of a lot of stuff, which itself is freeing. Moving confronts us with many challenges, like adjusting to new travel routes, meeting new people— all of which stimulate us and our brains, causing our dendrites to grow. Feel old and stuck in a rut—pack up and move!

Music

Making music brings people together, breaks down barriers, and generally leads to having a good time. Playing an instrument well—or even not so well—can make you feel young and exuberant again, like you're on top of the world. Playing a musical instrument exercises the brain and has been shown to increase

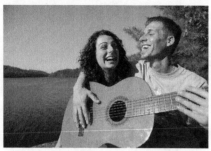

Playing music exercises the brain.

spatial-temporal reasoning, which is the foundation for success in math and science. Further evidence indicates that performing music increases reading ability.

Making music is a stress-reducer and helps to increase the performance of the immune system. Studies show that people who make music have higher levels of melatonin, a revitalized natural production of Human Growth Hormone. Older adults who make music show decreased levels of anxiety, depression and loneliness.

Listen to Music: You can change your mood faster with music than with drugs, except when injected intravenously. Step into a church and hear solemn music and you immediately feel pious, even inspired. Hear a funeral dirge and you feel somber. Listen to bee bop for a second or so and your toe will begin to tap on its own. Moving to an upbeat tune makes us feel light on our feet. We want to leap up and dance. We feel young and energetic. Soon endorphins, those feel-good hormones, are released into our brains and we do, indeed, feel youthful, full of vim and vigor.

Play a Musical Instrument: Playing a musical instrument exercises many interrelated dimensions of brain function, including listening, control of refined movements—sound and music, and uses sight to translate written notes into music. In addition to exercising the brain, playing a musical instrument draws us into the flow state—an altered state of consciousness where we feel "one with" what we're doing. Instead of playing an instrument, you become one with the music you and the instrument create. Learn to play a musical or take up an old one to bring more joy into your life—and those of your friends.

**It is the childlike mind that
find the kingdom.**

—Charles Fillmore

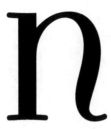

Naive

The naïve exhibit a lack of experience, understanding or sophistication. The naivety of youth is charming when they show unaffected simplicity of nature and an absence of artificiality. Youth tends to have a simple, unaffectedly direct style. The naive are unsuspecting, artless, guileless, candid, open, and plain. Jaded is boring and stuck. Embrace and enjoy being naïve.

Naked

In its exuberance youth often gets an urge to rip clothing off to dance naked in the sun. Being naked is pleasurable and fun and the youthful like doing what's fun. Youth loves to challenge taboos. They are daring and inclined to try new and unusual things. The youthful ignore how their bodies look. To be nude is to be free, to run free, to be open to nature, and to be ecstatic. It is healthful to expose all of our skin directly to sun, air, and water—wear sunscreen! Nudity creates openness, acceptance, love, and full enjoyment of nature. Get naked whenever you can.

Naughtiness

Engaging in harmless naughtiness is characteristic of the young—be it human or puppies. The young love to break the rules and to be mischievous. Mischief naughtiness is fun and feels good. Santa knows if you've been naughty or nice—he'll forgive you!

Nonconformity

Nonconformists do not conform to, and refuse to be bound by accepted beliefs, customs, or practices. They don't conform to generally accepted patterns of behavior or thought. Youth in its personal exploration often steps outside of accepted decorum and adopts an attitude dependent upon their own thoughts, independent from conventional or societal thought. Break out of rigid confines. You don't have to conform all the time.

Nootropics

Nootropics—also called smart drugs, memory enhancers, and cognitive enhancers—are foods and drugs that enhance cognition, memory, and learning. They are thought to work by altering the availability of the brain's supply of neurochemicals—neurotransmitters, enzymes, and hormones—or by improving the brain's oxygen supply or by stimulating nerve growth.

Popular nootropics include piracetam and racetams like pramiracetam, oxiracetam, and aniracetam. How racetams work is unknown. Racetams have been called "pharmacologically safe" drugs. Other substances sometimes classified as nootropics include hydergine, and vinpocetine. There are a variety of offshore anti-aging websites where a limited supply of nootropics can be imported for personal use.

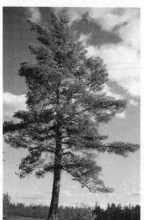

Nature is restorative.

Nature

Spending time outside in nature is relaxing, reduces stress, and is mentally restorative. The restorative effects of a natural environment, even if it is only a walk in the park, lead to renewed attention and positive emotions. One study

showed that after 45 minutes of taxing mental work, a walk out
of doors in nature lead to better recovery than did a walk in an
urban area. Merely looking at pictures of nature scenes (compared
to urban scenes) leads to an increased sense of well-being. Grab
opportunities to connect with nature. When walking or sitting
in a natural setting—a city park will do just fine—allow yourself
to slow down, drop your usual routines, and joyfully absorb the
influence of the place.

Nuts

Nuts are nature's perfect health food. They are high in fiber and
have lots of omega-3 fatty acids, which are essential for brain
health. Nuts are loaded with protein and they are full of antioxidant vitamins and minerals, which are important for scavenging
free radicals that cause disease and aging. Nuts are a great source
of B vitamins that are good for your heart and your brain. Nuts
are filled with healthy fats that benefit the elastin and collagen in
skin, helping to maintaining skin's structure and keep it resilient.

Nuts are a perfect snack. Small portions are advised because nuts
are high in calories. How-
ever, a nutrition study found
that even though being a
high-fat/high-cal food, nuts
don't promote weight gain
because they are so filling
that we tend to eat less of
them than other snacks. Add
a satisfying nutty crunch to
your salads with chopped
pecans or pistachios, which
have properties that brighten
and restore aging skin.

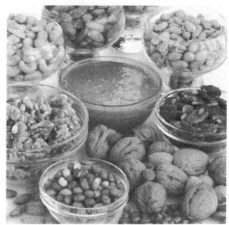

Nuts feed the brain.

Raw nuts are very high
in fiber; they are also a good source of vitamins and potassium, zinc,

iron, magnesium, copper and selenium. They control cholesterol level and strengthen your immune system. Raw nuts are good anti-aging food. Avoid salted and roasted nuts, which do more damage to your health than bring benefits.

Youthfulness is connected to the ability to see things new for the first time. So if your eyes still look at life with wonder, then you will seem young, even though you may not be chronologically young.

—Goldie Hawn

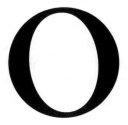

Olive Oil

Olive oil contains polyphenols, which are powerful antioxidants that help prevent age-related diseases. There are as many as 5 mg of antioxidant polyphenols in every 10 grams of olive oil. Polyphenols have been shown to reduce coronary artery disease and may be the substance involved in actually lowering blood pressure. In the early 1970s researchers concluded that the monounsaturated fats in olive oil were largely responsible for the low rates of heart disease and cancer among the peoples of Crete.

Olive oil is one of the finest sources you can use for delaying the aging process. Many age-related diseases and ailments are related to inflammation. Olive oil contains a natural anti-inflammatory ingredient, oleocanthal, which inhibits the activity of cyclooxygenase (COX). COX is present in nearly every aging person suffering from an inflammatory condition.

The polygene and oleic in olive oil are wonderful for your skin. Mix one egg and a tablespoon of olive oil and apply to dry and clean skin to promote a glowing and soft youthful-looking skin.

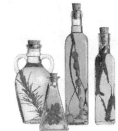

Secret of youthful skin.

Omega-3 Fatty Acids

Omega 3 fatty acids are poly-unsaturated fatty acids. Studies show that a diet rich in omega 3 fatty acids may help lower triglycerides and increase HDL cholesterol—the good cholesterol. Omega 3 fatty acids act as an anticoagulant to help prevent blood from clotting. Other studies show that these fatty acids help lower high blood pressure.

Omega-3s stave off dementia and Alzheimer's disease. Omega 3 anti-aging benefits are comprised from two forms of fatty acid: DHA and EPA. Research shows that people who regularly eat foods rich in omega-3 fatty acids do better on memory and cognition tasks. These fatty acids help quench the flames of chronic inflammation and act on an area of the brain that leads to improved mood and attitude among healthy people. Coldwater fish like salmon, tuna, trout, anchovies, and halibut are high in omega-3 fats, as are walnuts, pecans, almonds, flaxseed, kiwi fruits, and eggs.

Oysters

The expression "the world is my oyster", suggests that there's a world of benefits hidden inside their shell. Oysters, as we all know, are an aphrodisiac. So if you want to feel sexy and strut your stuff, eat up! However, if your mind wanders or you have memory lapses here and there, you may need more of the minerals zinc and iron in your diet. Hark! Oysters are rich in both iron and zinc. Low levels of iron and zinc are associated with poorer mental performance in children. These elements help keep grown-ups' minds sharp as well. Additionally, the high zinc content of oysters is a great beauty benefit as this mineral is a major player in skin renewal and repair. They helps create collagen, which provides the structural support in skin.

> Why, then, the world's mine oyster, which I with sword will open.
>
> —Pistol to Falstaff
> Shakespeare

Oatmeal

Oats are a good source of both soluble and insoluble fiber. Insoluble fiber has cancer-fighting properties because it attacks certain bile acids, reducing their toxicity. Research suggests that soluble fiber reduces LDL cholesterol without lowering HDL cholesterol. LDL is bad; HDL is good.

It has been found that those who regularly eat more oats are less likely to develop heart disease. Additionally, the phytochemicals in oats have cancer-fighting properties and are a good source of many nutrients including Vitamin E, zinc, selenium, copper, iron, manganese and magnesium. So eat up a big bowl of oatmeal whenever you can—especially on cold winter mornings.

Onion

Onions have antibacterial and antifungal properties and can kill worms and other parasites. Onions contain a number of compounds that help reduce cholesterol and blood pressure, and help prevent harmful blood clots. Eating onions can effectively improve lung and heart health and even reduce the risk for cancer. Legend has it that during the plague-epidemic in London, when the contagion spread everywhere, the owners of onion and garlic shops were the only persons who proved immune to the disease.

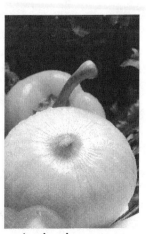

Anti-aging secret.

Sulfer-rich phytochemicals in onions give them their anti-aging benefits. Vigor, luster of the body and mental power increase with the use of onions. Onion-juice with honey taken daily in the morning for two to three weeks is believe to increase virility. The more "bite" in the bulb, the better.

Optimism

People with an optimistic outlook tend to have physical health according to findings by University of Pennsylvania researcher Martin Seligman, Ph.D., who showed that optimists have better immune activity than pessimists. Another study showed that optimism added an average of seven and a half years to life span. Research has found that an upbeat attitude—or happiness—lessens the burden of chronic pain from arthritis, and may reduce chances of developing cardiovascular disease. Happiness plays an important role in keeping your brain healthy and vital, too. Besides living longer, optimists suffer less stress. And optimists are more fun to be around than are pessimists. So practice looking at the glass as being half-full.

> You are as young as your faith, as old as your doubt; as young as your self-confidence, as old as your fear; as young as your hope, as old as your despair.
>
> —Douglas MacArthur

ORAC Score

A ORAC (Oxygen Radical Absorbance Capacity) score is used to measure the antioxidant strengths of food and other substances, with a higher score indicating that the food is better at protecting the body's cells from free radical-induced damage. The higher a food's ORAC score, the better that food is for you.

Eating foods containing at least 3,000 ORAC units a day is recommended. A half-cup of blueberries, for example, has 2,400 ORAC units. Dark-skinned vegetables and fruits have higher ORAC scores. Legumes rate highly. Be careful in comparing ORAC data. Make sure that the units and food compared are similar. Some evaluations compare ORAC units per grams dry weight, whereas others evaluate ORAC units wet weight and still others will look at ORAC units/serving.

Oxytocin

Oxytocin is a pituitary hormone that appears to be responsible for feelings of bonding and love. It is thought to trigger multi-orgasms in women and create firmer erections with increased ejaculate in men, which is why oxytocin has been dubbed by the media, "the love hormone".

Father Time is not always a hard parent, and, though he tarries for none of his children, often lays his hand lightly upon those who have used him well; making them old men and women inexorably enough, but leaving their hearts and spirits young and in full vigour. With such people the grey head is but the impression of the old fellow's hand in giving them his blessing, and every wrinkle but a notch in the quiet calendar of a well-spent life.

-Charles Dickens

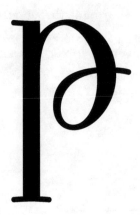

Passion Flower

Passion flower is a woody vine with pulpy fruit that grows in Argentina and Brazil. It is often used as an herbal alternative for soothing anxiety. Tea brewed from passion flower depresses the central nervous system and reduces spasms. It is believed that the combination of flavonoids in passion flower contribute to its effectiveness as an anxiolytic, which aids with relaxation, giving relief from occasional anxiety and panic resulting from stress. Compounds within passion flower have exhibited aphrodisiac, libido-enhancing and virility-enhancing properties in rats. Well, rats are like humans—physically— so it may be worth a try!

Pets

Living with a pet reduces the number of visits to the doctor, prolongs survival after a heart attack, and wards off depression. Sharing your home with a pet protects against a major problem of aging—high blood pressure. Pets boost survival rates for coronary care unit patients, one study showed.

Keeping a pet in a house is an opportunity to enjoy the benefits of touching. Touch therapy is said to be very effective in relaxing and making one feel stress free. One study showed that when pet-owning stockbrokers with high blood pressure were faced with mental stress, their blood pressure increased less than half as

much as in their counterparts who had
no pet pals. When a person interacts
with a pet, the central nervous system
releases hormones that cause feelings
of pleasure—including oxytocin.

Pets bring out your inner child.
Romping with your dog and tickling
your cat can be very refreshing. Pets
are caring and giving. Hop on down
to the animal shelter and bring home
a furry friend.

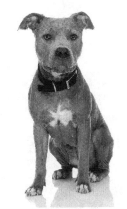

People with pets live longer.

Phosphatidylserine

Phosphatidylserine's primary benefit is to increase cognitive
function and long term memory. It is a phospholipid, a fat found
throughout the body's cells, particularly in the brain. It is an essential component of brain cell membranes and has very significant effects on memory, brain longevity and mood. It is essential
to the functioning of all cells in the body. It maintains the flexibility and fluidity of cell membranes to maximize the absorption
of nutrients.

Phytonutrients

Phytonutrients—pronounced "fight-o-nutrients" and also called
phytochemicals—are natural bioactive compounds found in fruits,
vegetables and their juices. More than 900 different phytonutrients
have been discovered so far in plant foods and more will be identified
and researched in the future.

Most phytochemicals have antioxidant activity and protect
our cells against oxidative damage and reduce the risk of developing certain types of cancer. Phytochemicals with antioxidant
activity include allyl sulfides in onions, leeks, and garlic, carotenoids in fruits and carrots, flavonoids in fruits and vegetables,
polyphenols in tea and grapes. Isoflavones, found in soy, imitate
human estrogens and help to reduce menopausal symptoms and
osteoporosis. Indoles, which are found in cabbages, stimulate

enzymes that make the estrogen less effective and could reduce the risk for breast cancer. Other phytochemicals, which interfere with enzymes, are protease inhibitors—soy and beans, terpenes—citrus fruits and cherries.

Saponins found in beans interfere with the replication of cell DNA, thereby preventing the multiplication of cancer cells. Capsaicin, found in hot peppers, protects DNA from carcinogens. The phytochemical allicin from garlic has anti-bacterial properties. Some phytochemicals bind physically to cell walls thereby preventing the adhesion of pathogens to human cell walls. Proanthocyanidins are responsible for the anti-adhesion properties of cranberry. Consumption of cranberries will reduce the risk of urinary tract infections and will improve dental health.

Piracetam

Piracetam is a nootropic or "smart drug" that regulates brain function and slows brain aging. It improves communication between the two hemispheres of the brain. Piracetam stimulates the cholinergic system in the cerebral cortex to speed up metabolism and promotes the synthesis of ATP. Using piracetam improves short-term memory and overall cognitive functioning, including increased cellular protein synthesis and inter-hemispheric and intercellular communication.

Piracetam helps to prevent and correct memory losses due to old age, sharpening memory, relieving boredom and improving clarity and attention to detail. It improves brain function and stimulates the central nervous system without any toxicity or addictive properties. Its effects are increased when taken with DMAE, centrophenoxine, coline, or hydergine.

Piracetam is often used without medical supervision as an anti-aging treatment, which is ill-advised by medical practitioners. While no toxic side effects have been reported it reacts synergistically with DMAE, centrophenoxine, choline, Deaner, lecithin, and hydergine, requiring lower doses of each. The Federal Drug Administration has not approved the use of piracetam in the United States although it can be ordered online from Europe.

Play

We think of play as something that children do. Play is a state of mind—finding enjoyment and fun in small things, love of life. Playing gives us a chance to be silly, to make mistakes, to get outside of ourselves, to connect with our "inner" child. We feel "alive" when playing. Laughter often accompanies play. When playing we may break rules and try new things, which can help to get out of "rut" thinking to a creative break-through. Playing exercises the heart, reducing the risk of hypertension and heart attacks. Play can enhance your energy level. In short, playing brings back youthful exuberance.

Popcorn

Corn has the highest level of anti-oxidants of any grain or vegetable. A typical six-cup bag of microwave popcorn delivers almost 25 percent of the recommended daily intake of fiber for about 200 calories or less. If you are an emotional eater, eat unbuttered popcorn. Popcorn can be flavored with garlic-flavored olive oil instead of butter. Pop in that DVD, roast up some popcorn and have a great evening.

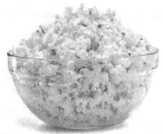

Popcorn is a healthy snack.

Positive Thinking

Negative and judgmental thinking wears us down. We doubt ourselves, self-confidence falls and immune system weakens. We withdraw and resist taking risks—we act and feel "old". Positive thinking—being optimistic, on the other hand, decreases risk of heart attacks and increases longevity. People who live long lives generally have a positive attitude. Researchers believe that positive thinking stimulates the immune system, making us more resilient to illness. Research conducted at Yale showed that people with positive attitude lived on the average of 7.5 years longer than those with pessimistic attitudes.

> The day a person becomes a cynic is the day he loses his youth.
> — Marvin D. Levy

Negative thinking is rooted in habitual ways of looking at the world—the half empty glass. Like any other bad habit, habitual pessimism can be changed—but it does take work because negative thinking is entrenched and circular. One technique is to catch yourself telling yourself something negative, like "I'll never get ahead" or "people just can't be trusted", for example. Write the negative thought down, word-for-word. Then objectively challenge the thought that you were saying to yourself. Ask, "Is this true?" "Is it true that I will never get ahead? Is it true that I will never make any progress in my career?" Ask, "Is it true that no one can ever be trusted?" "Is it true that I cannot trust anyone?" Of course the statements are extreme overgeneralizations.

Next, rewrite the negative statement into a "true" statement that is positive or at least neutral. Make sure to write out the alternative statement. "Getting ahead is hard because there are hurtles I must overcome." Or "Some people can be trusted and some can not." Next, when you catch yourself telling yourself the "false" negative statement, yell, "Stop!" loudly in your mind and deliberately switch to thinking the alternative "true" statement.

The more that you identify your specific negative "self-talk" and replace it with neutral or positive self-talk, the more optimistic your outlook will become. It will take discipline on your part, but you can "reprogram" your mental scripts. As you do you will fell more empowered and in control of your life.

Power lifting & Bodybuilding

Powerlifting and bodybuilding slows down the process of bone deterioration from osteoporosis in both men and women. The sport encourages socializing and making new friends, and improved self-esteem from striving for performance goals. Powerlifting and bodybuilding extends youthfulness through generating muscle tone, and strength, developing a healthy lifestyle. Bodybuilding enthusiasts learn what is good for the body, which develops better eating habits and healthier nutritional eating habits. Usually supplements are included—vitamins, minerals, protein powders, and amino acids—which replenish and rejuvenate the body.

Pranks

Pranks are practical jokes or stunts to purposely make someone feel foolish or victimized. They are typically lighthearted and a tease. Pranks were a common feature of ancient seasonal festivals. During Saturnalia, a Roman winter celebration, participants would dance, drink and play jokes on each other; slaves pretended to rule their masters, and a mock king, the Lord of Misrule, reigned for a day. Court jesters often played tricks on kings and courtiers. Generally pranks are the work of youth—just for the fun of it. Halloween and April Fool's Day are two prankster holidays.

Pray

Praying relieves stress, reduces anxiety, and promotes calm in the midst of a storm. Regular praying stabilizes mood, giving a feeling of well-being. Praying builds faith—trust—trust in the unknown, trust in the spiritual power of the universe—wonder. Youth is naturally trusting. Sometimes it is called being gullible, naïve. Praying brings back this openness and willingness to trust. Where oldsters approach with skepticism; the youthful embrace with openness and trust.

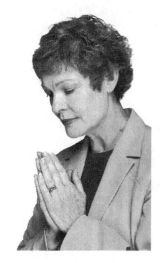

Praying soothes worry and anxiety. Worry is us talking to ourselves about problems and potential perils. Worry triggers anxiety and anxiety triggers worry, setting up a vicious cycle that robs us of sleep and fun.

Praying is soothing.

Importantly, however, we can only have one thought or image in the mind at a time. You can use this principle to crowd out worry. Praying involves saying the words of the prayer or mantra. You can quiet your worry by crowding it out with the prayer, where we substitute the words of the prayer for the words of the worry. Some people also use a rosary or worry beads, which are similar. When holding the first bead, say the "Hail Mary", mantra, or other prayer. Then move to the second bead while saying the prayer or mantra. In this praying ritual" you use thinking and moving your fingers to crowd the worrying thoughts out.

When praying, negative worries are replaced with the soothing words of the prayer, which promotes a more encouraging outlook on life and the world. Praying increases focus and attention and clears the mind of distractions and negative thoughts. With decreased anxiety and fear, we sleep better—like a baby.

Produce—Fruits and Vegetables

Eating large helpings of fruits and vegetables keeps weight down—we all know that! But studies also show that certain produce can provide surprising anti-aging benefits. Berries, especially blueberries, have powerful memory-boosting potential. Berries combat free radicals, molecules that can cause widespread cell damage and are linked to chronic inflammation. Inflammation is thought to be at the root of most chronic diseases, from cancer, heart disease, and diabetes to Alzheimer's, arthritis, osteoporosis, and aging in general. Furthermore, berries are chock-full of Vitamin C, another potent antioxidant that helps to keep skin complexion looking smooth and youthful by fighting skin-damaging free radicals.

Eating spinach and other dark leafy greens helps to keep vision sharp because they are a prime source of lutein and zeaxanthin, plant pigments that protect eyes from the harmful effects of ultraviolet light. Leafy greens are also rich in Vitamin K, which plays a role in reducing bone loss that leads to fractures in the aging.

Propolis

Propolis is resin from tree bark and leaves gathered by honeybees, who combine it with nectar, creating a mix of wax, pollen and bee bread. Bees use propolis to seal their hives, protecting it from outside contaminants and to sterilize themselves as they come and go from the hive. Propolis contains a natural antibiotic and has been used since antiquity to heal sores and ulcers, internally and externally. Synthetic antibiotics, like penicillin, carry with them side effects, whereas propolis is a natural antibiotic that has no such side effects. Propolis is also packed with beneficial nutrients. It contains 500 more bioflavonoids—Vitamin P—than found in oranges. Except for Vitamin K, propolis has all the known all minerals required by the body except sulfur.

Puzzles

Mind games are a great way to stay involved and engaged in the world. Games can exercise different parts of your mind and entice your curiosity. Choose social games like chess or bridge that exercise your brain while keeping you connected with others.

> **Mere longevity is a good thing for those who watch Life from the side lines. For those who play the game, an hour may be a year, a single day's work an achievement for eternity.**
>
> —Helen Hayes

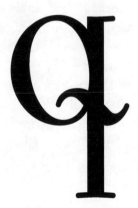

Quality Time

Quality time is time spent with family and friends that is important, special, productive, creative or profitable. It is time that is set
aside for giving the person at hand undivided attention. During
quality time we build bonds, enjoy sharing emotional support.
Besides having fun, quality time is rejuvenating—it relieves stress,
and strengthens immune system. Make a list of people in your
life in whose company you feel more alive, happy, and optimistic.
Make an effort to spend more time with them.

Question

Students of all ages use questions in learning. The Socratic
method of questioning
student responses may
be used by a teacher to
indirectly lead students
toward the truth to
help them form logical
conclusions.

Questions can be used as
icebreakers as a way to start
up a conversation and meet
new people. Questions that

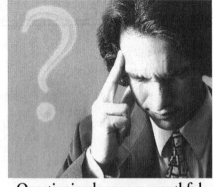

Questioning keeps you youthful.

make you think can be entertaining starters for a discussion or a meeting. Questions can serve as icebreaker in formal or informal gatherings. They can invite interest and serve as thoughtful stress busters. Questions that make you think can spice up your get-to-gethers. Silly questions can create humor. Such questions can be fun. Some serious, yet, interesting questions that make you think can give a witty touch to your gatherings. Be it a business meeting or an informal get-together, questions making you think are great options to break ice.

Question Authority: Benjamin Franklin was often quoted as saying "it is the first responsibility of every citizen to question authority." Patriots help to keep government in check by questioning its authority. Youth is well known for challenging authority on just about every issue. Get in touch with your power and question authority.

People grow old only by deserting their ideals. Years may wrinkle the skin, but to give up interest wrinkles the soul. You are as young as your faith, as old as your doubt; as young as your self-confidence, as old as your fear; as young as your hope as old as your despair. In the central place of every heart there is a recording chamber. So long as it receives messages of beauty, hope, cheer and courage, so long are you young. When your heart is covered with the snows of pessimism and the ice of cynicism, then, and then only, are you grown old. And then, indeed as the ballad says, you just fade away.

—Douglas MacArthur

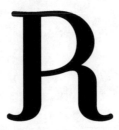

Random Acts of Kindness

When you perform an act of kindness, such as helping someone or smiling at someone or doing something nice for someone, you get healthful benefits, according to Dr. Wayne Dyer. It makes you feel good. Chemicals react and the body feels pleasure. Dyer said "…beneficial effects of kindness on the immune system and the increased production of serotonin have been proven. Conversely, unkindness weakens the body and puts us into a state of dissonance. So extend acts of kindness; ask for nothing in return."

View every human encounter as a "holy relationship" with the ability to celebrate and honor others, no matter who. When you do something kind for someone else, their brain releases serotonin—and so does yours! Serotonin is a hormone that makes us feel good. So, every act of kindness yields two happier people. Extend good will, care and consideration, which is instrumental in inspiring hope in others.

Rapamycin

Scientists have discovered Easter Island 'fountain of youth' drug can extend life by ten years. In tests, the anti-aging pill increased the life expectancy of animals by thirty-eight percent. Scientists are now looking at its benefits for humans. The chemical is produced by a microbe that lives in the Easter Island soil, which suppresses the immune system and makes patients vulnerable to viruses and bacteria.

Rapamycin is a drug used to keep the body from rejecting organ and bone marrow transplants. It blocks certain white blood cells that can reject foreign tissues and organs and also blocks a protein that is involved in cell division. Rapamycin is a type of antibiotic—an immunosuppressant, and a type of serine/threonine kinase inhibitor. Rapamycin is now called sirolimus. The life extension possibilities of rapamycin are in the early stages of research and still speculative. Research has shown an increase life span of mice by about thirty percent. It suppresses the immune system and healthy people should never use it in an attempt to extend life. This could be risky. Still, researchers are excited about the possibilities.

In the study, reported in the journal *Nature*, scientists tested rapamycin on nearly 2,000 laboratory mice aged around 600 days, roughly the equivalent to a 60-year-old person. Around a quarter of the mice were given a normal diet, the others the Easter Island chemical. From the point the mice began the treatment, the drug extended the females' life expectancy by 38 percent, and males by 28 percent. Overall it expanded their life span by 9 to 14 percent. Repeated studies have shown that cutting calories can make animals and people live longer. Experts believe that rapamycin, which acts on a protein in cells called TOR, might fool the body into thinking that calories are being restricted.

Red Wine

The French have a relatively low incidence of coronary heart disease, despite having a diet rich in saturated fats. This observation lead to coining the term, "The French Paradox", in 1992 which refers to France's high red wine consumption is a primary factor in keeping heart disease low. Research suggests that moderate drinkers are less likely to suffer heart attacks than are abstainers or heavy drinkers. Red wine is packed with resveratrol, an antioxidant, which works to protect the body against the effects of aging.

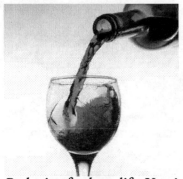

Red wine for long life. Yum!

One or two glasses of red wine a day can help keep your body young. Animal research suggests that high amounts of resveratrol may counteract cell death in the heart and brain, which could mean this compound has even greater potential to prolong life. Don't over do it. Limit yourself to one five-ounce glass a day.

Reflexology

Reflexology is a holistic therapy that activates the body's ability to heal itself by using a specific pressure technique on points of the feet and hands. It strengthens the immune system, detoxifies the body and allows a state of total relaxation. Reflexology can be used to treat acute and chronic conditions such as hormonal imbalances, stress related conditions, back pain, arthritis, sports injures, digestive disorders and infertility.

Relax

Relaxation is the opposite of stress. While stress brings harmful health effects, relaxation helps our bodies to rest, heal and function better. By practicing daily relaxation techniques, you can train yourself to turn off your stress and replace it with calm energy. This will improve your blood pressure, heart rate and ability to cope with life's challenges.

Relationships

Relationships are an important part of health. Not only do strong bonds with other people mean you will have help when you need it, being connected also means protection from loneliness, depression, and mental illness. Spend time cultivating your relationships with friends and family to improve your health and the quality of your life.

Resilience

Resilience doesn't make problems go away. It is the ability to roll with the punches. It is the capacity to cope with stress and catastrophe. When something goes wrong, resilient people bounce back. People who lack resilience dwell on problems, feel victimized, become overwhelmed and turn to unhealthy coping mechanisms, such as substance abuse.

You build resilience by getting connected and building strong, positive relationships with family and friends, who provide support and acceptance. Develop a sense of purpose for your life to have something meaningful to focus on can help you share emotions, feel gratitude and experience an enhanced sense of well-being. Laugh. Humor is a helpful coping mechanism. If you can't find any humor in a situation, turn to other sources for a laugh, such as a funny book or movie. Learn from experience. Build on skills and strategies that helped you through the rough times, and don't repeat those that didn't help.

Remain hopeful. Find something in each day that signals a change for the better. Be optimistic and expect good results. Take care of yourself. Participate in activities and hobbies you enjoy, exercising regularly, getting plenty of sleep and eating well. Keep a journal. Journaling helps to see situations in a new way and to identify patterns in your behavior and reactions.

Accept and anticipate change. Expecting changes to occur makes it easier to adapt to them, tolerate them and even welcome them. Work toward a goal. Do something every day that gives you a sense of accomplishment. Take action. Figure out what needs to be done, make a plan and take action. Maintain perspective. Look at your situation in the larger context of your life and of the world. Practice stress management and relaxation techniques. Restore an inner sense of peace and calm by practicing such stress-management and relaxation techniques as yoga, meditation, deep breathing, visualization, imagery, prayer or muscle relaxation.

When adversity strikes, you still experience anger, grief and pain, but you're able to go on with daily tasks, remain generally

optimistic and go on with your life. Being resilient also doesn't
mean being stoic or going it alone. In fact, being able to reach out
to others for support is a key component of resilience.

Resveratrol

Resveratrol is a phytonutrient that is produced when certain
plants are under attack by pathogens like bacteria and fungi.
Researchers have shown that resveratrol extends the life span of
yeasts, mice, and certain short-lived fish. A Harvard research
group shed light on the process by which resveratrol significantly
improves health and lifespan in mice. In so doing, The Harvard
group discovered what may be the universal cause of aging. They
contend that this occurs when a specialized dual-role enzyme
known as SIRT1 shifts its attention, from keeping genetic peace
by guarding and regulating, which genes are switched on and
off in a cell, to repairing double-strand DNA breaks caused by
oxidative warfare. The essential discovery is paradoxical. When
SIRT1 repeatedly rushes to fight DNA damage in the name of
inhibiting aging, some of the genes it has formerly guarded express
themselves in ways that are inimical to the integrity of the cell.
The result is an acceleration of the aging process.

This understanding suggests new ways to halt or reverse
age-related disease, through the use of natural sirtuin activators,
such as resveratrol found in red wine. While aging still remains a
mystery to be solved, the new research allows important pieces of
the puzzle to fall into place and goes a long way toward unveiling
what may be thought of as the secrets of aging.

Youth is wasted on the young.

—George Bernard Shaw

Reverse Biological Age

1. Change your perceptions.
2. Deep rest, restful awareness, and restful sleep.
3. Lovingly nurture you body through healthy food.
4. Use nutritional complements wisely.
5. Enhance mind/body integration: breathing exercises, yoga, tai chi, qigong, aikido, etc.
6. Exercise: strength and aerobic conditioning.
7. Eliminate toxins from you life.
8. Cultivate flexibility and creativity in consciousness.
9. Love and loving relationships.
10. Maintain a youthful mind.

—**Deepak Chopra, M.D. & David Simon, M.D.**
Grow Younger, Live Longer
Ten Steps to Reverse Aging

Rosemary

The pine-like leaves of rosemary are perforated with oil glands and the extracts contain flavonoids and compounds including carnosol and carsonic acid that help protect the body cells against the oxidative stresses caused by free radicals and toxins that lead to aging. Hydrating and oxygenating moisturizer with rosemary fights free radical damage, protects, nourishes and energizes skin. Vitamin B complex helps provide increased oxygenation and circulation for your complexion.

Rosemary has antibacterial, antiseptic, antispasmodic and analgesic—pain relieving—properties. Rosemary extracts or diluted rosemary oil was used for thousands of years as a salve to be applied externally on painful muscles and joints stiffened by rheumatism. Added to bath water, it provides a relaxing soak that eases pain and stimulates blood flow.

Royal Jelly

Royal jelly is tasty honey-sweet substance secreted from the salivary glands of worker bees that serves as food for all young larvae and as the only food for larvae that will develop into queen bees. Royal jelly contains all the B-vitamins, vitamins A, C, D, E and K, more than a dozen key minerals, 18 amino acids, and other important constituents, including nucleic acids (DNA and RNA). Adenosine triphosphate (ATP), adenosine diphosphate (ADP) and adenosine monophosphate (AMP) are also found in Royal Jelly.

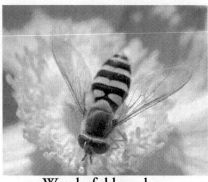

Wonderful busy bee.

A study in mice showed royal jelly given for 16 weeks helped them live longer. Rodent studies also indicate that royal jelly has beneficial effects on bone strength. Whether royal jelly has longevity benefits in humans is not known—but many believe that it does. And it is definitely yummy!

Nobody grows old merely by living a number of years. We grow old by deserting our ideals. Years may wrinkle the skin, but to give up enthusiasm wrinkles the soul.

~Samuel Ullman

S

Sea Moss

Sea moss is a red algae that grows along the rocky part of the Atlantic coast. Sea moss is mainly comprised of carrageenan, which is used as a thickener and stabilizer. It has anti-aging qualities and is a known aphrodisiac and fertility enhancer and contains high concentrate of calcium, iodine, sulfur, potassium, and Vitamins A, D, E, F and K.

Sea moss is an antioxidant that speeds up cellular repair and diminishes signs of aging. Grind up dry sea moss in a food processor and sprinkle it on food. When soaked in water, sea moss retains it's gelatinous form and can be blended into smoothies, shakes. For a little extra zing in the bedroom, try sea moss.

Skip

Skipping is a style of gait movement involving a combination of walking and jumping. It is a hippity hoppity gait that comes naturally to children. It expresses joy in movement.

Skipping is great for fitness, agility, coordination and general health. Two to five minutes of skipping every day helps prevent osteoporosis. Skipping combines the skills of rhythm and timing. Skipping is a wonderful workout for both the heart and lungs, and it works the muscles, too. To feel light, nimble and young—skip! It's fun.

Follow the Yellow Brick Road

Follow the Yellow Brick Road.
Follow, follow, follow, follow,
Follow the Yellow Brick Road.
Follow the Yellow Brick, Follow the Yellow Brick,
Follow the Yellow Brick Road.

We're off to see the Wizard, The Wonderful Wizard of Oz.
You'll find he is a whiz of a Wiz! If ever a Wiz! there was.
If ever oh ever a Wiz! there was The Wizard of Oz is one because,
Because, because, because, because, because.
Because of the wonderful things he does.

—Dorothy
The Wizard of Oz

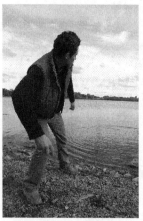

Youthful pastime.

Skip Stones

Stone skipping is a pastime, which involves throwing a stone with a flattened surface across a lake or other body of water in such a way that it bounces along the surface of the water. The object of the game is to see how many times a stone can be made to bounce before sinking.

Sardines

Sardines are budget-friendly fatty-fish that contain omega-3 fatty acids, which are thought to be instrumental in maintaining brain function from early development throughout life. DHA, an omega-3, is present in the brain, so having those good-for-you omega-3s in your diet is thought to boost brain function. The fatty acids in fish go straight to the synapses of nerve cells, so they play an important role in how neurons communicate with one another, which may have a positive affect throughout life on learning and memory.

Self-Hypnosis

Hypnosis is an effective tool for changing attitude and behavior. "You are only as old as you feel," goes the popular saying. If you want to look and feel younger you must first get past the cultural brainwashing that paints a picture of an inevitable decline with age, over which you have no control.

Set a positive intention to actually do something constructive along the lines of exercise, diet and proper hydration. Being able to enter a relaxed state of mind and body on a regular basis can actually reduce the wear and tear on your cells. The relaxation that accompanies hypnosis can enable you to enter this type of restorative state at will. Hypnosis and self-hypnosis have the added advantage in that you can also reprogram the behaviors and attitudes needed for a more youthful state while you relax.

Selenium

Selenium salts are toxic in large amounts, but trace amounts of the element are necessary for cellular function. Selenium helps to block cancer and reduces heart disease. It relieves stress and anxiety. It prevents mutations, repairs cells, and boosts immune functions. Selenium works with Vitamin E in protecting against free radicals. Selenium is found in grains, sunflower seeds, meat, seafood, and garlic. High levels are found in kidney, tuna, crab, lobster, and Brazil nuts.

Service

Being of service is an integral part of the journey toward finding fulfillment. Think of a time when you participated in making someone's life better. How do you feel recalling your service to another? Most people say that it feels good when they did something meaningful, something that mattered. Being of service to others takes our focus off of ourselves and looks for how we might be useful where and how we are. When we feel grateful, we naturally want to share ourselves and our good fortune. Being of service increases our gratitude and joy and our experience of the unity of all life.

Sex

Research has revealed that regular sexual activity with one partner extends life expectancy by at least two years. Almost all healthy long-lived people stay married and enjoy regular lovemaking until the end of their days. As they say—use it or lose it!

Sex and touching are thought to be essential parts of health. Sex releases an assortment of beneficial chemicals in the body. Sex and touching help us bond with others, strengthens relationships, and increases our sense of self-worth. Frequent sex may even extend your life by years.

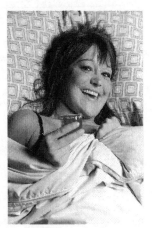

Sexual intercourse is more than just exercise. There are numerous health benefits to love-making. Many are the same as non-physical expressions of love, but stronger. Simply being in love increases your DHEA levels. Men who had sex at least twice a week were half as likely to die as men who had sex less than once a month. Emotional intimacy during sex eases stress and fosters an overall sense of

Use it or lose it.

well-being. Making love can help keep you looking good, too. A British study reported that couples with a healthy sex life can look up to seven years younger than those who aren't as intimate. It seems that sex reduces external signs of aging caused by stress.

Silliness

When acting silly we feel like kids again. Being silly is rejuvenating. Notice how young children so love giggling and being silly. When we're silly endorphins—the body's own feel-good drug— are released in our brain. Being silly feels good. Lighten up and stop being so serious. Wear a goofy hat. Make a funny face when having your picture taken and carry it in your wallet or post it on your frig to remind you to be silly. Find opportunities to giggle. Be playful. Notice the folly in things. Find ways to make jokes about serious happenings.

Silver

Silver is one of the oldest infection fighters known and was used long before antibiotics were developed. Silver can kill hundreds of different disease organisms, including bacteria, fungi, yeasts, viruses and parasites. Colloidal silver is a metallic silver in a solvent—usually water. Available over the counter, pure colloidal silver is widely accepted as a gargle for tonsillitis, sore throats, gingivitis, and as an anti-septic for psoriasis, cuts and abrasion, and for treating internal infections such as ring-worm. It is important to always use only pure (ion-free) silver protein.

Skin Care

Regular cleansing is very important to keep skin free from dirt and dead cells. Cleaning the skin with natural scrubs removes dead cells and adds a glow to the skin. Proper toning and moisturizing using natural toner and cream keeps the skin soft and clean. The cleaning regimen followed dedicatedly, is an antiaging process in itself. It is important to keep skin clean from pollution, harmful UV rays and other external impurities. Wear sunscreen to help prevent sun damage and premature skin aging. Drink eight or nine glasses of water everyday to keep your skin hydrated and nice and plump. When your skin is clean and radiant you slow skin aging, look healthy, and feel youthful.

Skinny Dipping

Skinny dipping or swimming nude, usually in unheated water, is mischievous with an element of sexual rebelliousness to it, though sexual activity does not necessarily take place. Throwing off your clothes and diving into a pool or pond with your friends is a lotta fun. But be a little careful because public nudity is illegal in some places. Skinny dipping is best at a private swimming pool to avoid getting ticketed.

Sky Diving

Former President George H. W. Bush celebrated his 75th, 80th, and 85th birthdays by skydiving. The 41st president said. "You don't want to sit around, just because you're an old guy, drooling in the corner." An adrenaline rush definitely makes us feel alive and feeling alive is being youthful.

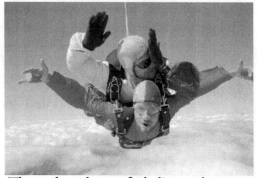

The rush makes us feel alive and young.

Sleep

Sleep is important for concentration, memory formation and the repair of damage to your body's cells during the day. Researchers believe that during sleep, neurons can shut down and repair any damage done during the day. Without these repairs, the neurons may not function correctly due to a buildup of waste products.

Sleep is important for the formation of memories. Chronic lack of sleep increases the risk for developing obesity, diabetes, cardiovascular disease and infections. In research studies, rats normally live two to three years, but if rats are totally deprived of sleep, they only live about five weeks. They also develop sores; their immune systems do not work well and their body temperature drops. Humans deprived of sleep for long periods begin hallucinating and develop other mental problems.

Sleep helps repair body and keeps the heart healthy. Sleep reduces stress and improves memory. Sleep is restorative. Rest and sleep provide an opportunity for the body to cleanse, repair, and rejuvenate on a deep cellular level.

Snuggle and Cuddle

Physical touch is actually good for the body because soothes, comforts, and relaxes. The body heals faster when stress is relieved, anxiety is minimized, and hope replaces fear. We all know how good it feels to be cuddled after a long day at work, having reassuring arms around you to let you know you're loved.

Simple things like cuddling, or holding hands whenever you go out, are ways to show your love. Massaging is a good way to relieve the tension in your body. Give your partner massages, perhaps while the both of you are watching TV, or just before bedtime. It doesn't have to be a full body massage; it could be just the head, neck and shoulders.

Smell the Flowers

How many times have you wished for more hours in your day? Stopping to smell the flowers has a time-expanding effect. Slowing down to enjoy the small beauties and delights, encourages us to live more fully in the here and now. We live in the moment, not in the past or the future. Practice appreciating the moment.

Smell The Flowers

As the Seeker and the Shaman Woman sat in a garden on a beautiful day the Shaman Woman noticed that the Seeker was frowning and staring distractedly into the distance.

"Is something troubling you?" asked the Shaman Woman.

"How can I enjoy my life when I know that sooner or later I'm going to die?" the Seeker lamented.

As the Shaman Woman listened she leaned over, picked a nearby lilac sprig and passed it slowly by the Seeker's nose. "Ah," the Seeker sighed, his frown dissolving into a smile.

"Humm," the Shaman nodded, "always remember to stop and smell the flowers."

-Beverly A. Potter
The Worrywart's Companion

Smile

The brain does not make a distinction between reality and pretense. Pretend to feel a certain way and soon you actually *do* feel that way because the brain produces the chemicals to match what you are thinking. Stop reading and smile for a moment—*really* smile. Grin from ear to ear. Feels good, doesn't it.

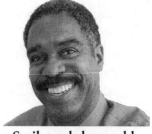

Smile and the world smiles back!

In *Peak Performance*, Dr. Charles Garfield describes how he noticed that when athletes lifted weights to exhaustion, they usually grimaced at the painful effort. In an experiment, Garfield instructed the athletes to smile when they got to the point of exhaustion. Interestingly, when smiling the weight-lifers were able to add two to three more reps to their performance.

Smiling tells your brain that you feel enthusiastic and in response your brain releases feel-good chemicals into your bloodstream so that you soon actually *do* feel good. Practice smiling.

> When you're smilin' keep on smilin'
> The whole world smiles with you
> And when you're laughin' oh when you're laughin'
> The sun comes shinin' through
> But when you're cryin' you bring on the rain
> So stop your sighin' 'be happy again
>
> —Louis Armstrong

Smiling is a great way to change your attitude, connect with people and give benefit to your body. Like relaxation, smiling counteracts the effects of stress. By forcing ourselves to smile, we "trick" the body into believing that everything is good, thereby reducing stress. Like a switch, smiling can actually change your mood. So put a smile on, even if you don't feel like it, and pretty soon you'll be smiling for real.

Remind yourself to smile more often. Smile as soon as you wake up and often throughout the day. Smiling will make you look more attractive and inviting. It will change your mood. Smile. Smile. Smile.

Socialize

Socializing is rejuvenating. Research shows that people with strong social support systems go to the hospital less often and live longer. Sharing thoughts, discussing problems and smiling together lowers stress. Older people, especially if they have lost their spouse, can get isolated. Making friends was practically effortless when in college, but becomes a challenge as we age. If you like to read, joining a book discussion group at your library is a wonderful meeting point for making friends with like-minded people. Take classes at your local college. Not only will you exercise your brain with learning something new, but you will have a chance to rub shoulders with potential friends. Join a health club. Volunteering is a traditional way to get out, do something of service, and to meet people. You might even try on-line dating. Nothing ventured; nothing gained.

Spending time with family and friends builds a strong support network and prevents loneliness. Plus, quality time with friends or family provides an additional source of activity, whether you partake in intellectual endeavors, physical activities, or volunteer pursuits.

Solitude

Solitude is not a state of loneliness or undesired isolation. It is a state of being with self. Solitude is not a boring state, a state of negative mentality, a state of pain. Solitude is a kind of voluntary retreat or retirement. It is surprisingly relaxing and provides the calm for reflection. Solitude can improve energy level, increase self confidence and tends to support a strong positive attitude towards life. Enjoying solitude everyday for a few moments is not only a good way to relax but also an easy way to charge battery of life, with inspiration, motivation and positive thoughts.

Soya

Soya helps to maintain estrogen levels in women in their menopausal years. Soya helps to alleviate menopausal hot flush and
protect against Alzheimer's disease, osteoporosis and heart disease.
Fermented soya products are more easily digested, so are more nutritional without causing food intolerances. Unlike soya, soy sauce
is full of salt and should be used sparingly, if at all.

Soy Beans

Soy beans are a low-fat, no-cholesterol food full of beneficial nutrients, including plenty of protein, both soluble fiber. It is good for
your heart, and insoluble fiber, which speeds intestinal elimination,
as well as a wealth of vitamins and minerals including B vitamins,
calcium, iron, magnesium and zinc. Soy has an abundance of phytochemicals such as flavonoids, phytates, phytosterols, polyphenols,
terpenes and saponins. Soy has anticancer characteristics. It slows
benign prostate enlargement and breast cancer.

Soy helps fight heart disease and slows osteoporosis, a disease
of aging, which weakens bones, due to the fact that soy offers
abundant calcium in a form the body readily absorbs. Soy can be
eaten as soybeans, tofu, soy sauce, miso, soy oil, soymilk, soy flour
and textured soy protein is put into drinks.

Spirulina

Blue-green, fresh water algae is considered by many to be the
worlds most perfect food. Rich in protein, vitamins, minerals, and
carotenoids—a type of antioxidant that can help protect cells from
damage. It contains nutrients, including B complex vitamins,
beta-carotene, Vitamin E, manganese, zinc, copper, iron, selenium, and gamma linolenic acid—an essential fatty acid. Adding
spirulina to cultured immune system cells significantly increases
the production of infection fighting cytokines, say immunologists
at UC Davis School of Medicine and Medical Center.

Nutrient packed spirulina is an ideal anti-aging food for older
people who do not eat much, eat inappropriately, or cannot ab-

sorb enough nutrients. It is ninety-five percent digestible because it has soft cell walls. Small amounts can help balance and stabilise the immune system, freeing up more of our metabolic energy for vitality, healing and assimilation of nutrients. Complex sugars from spirulina have been shown to increase antibody production and infection fighting T-cells. Mice have shown increased immunity, bone marrow reproduction, growth of thymus and spleen when fed complex sugars and phycocyanin from spirulina.

Spinach

Spinach is a versatile, affordable, readily available, low-calorie leafy green vegetable that is loaded with beauty-enhancing nutrients, including lutein, which keeps your eyes healthy and bright. Spinach also contains a significant amount of beta-carotene, as well as Vitamin C, several B vitamins, magnesium, iron, calcium, potassium, zinc, dietary fiber, and even omega-3 fatty acids, making it a wonderfully nutrient-dense vegetable.

Spontaneity

Being spontaneous as a person is defined as having an open, natural, and uninhibited manner. As we age we tend to get struck in a rut, rarely spontaneous, always following the same routine. Being open to change can be a good thing. The mysterious is beautiful. The unknown, unplanned, and spontaneous are beautiful. You cannot control every detail of what happens. So simply go along with it. This produces a childlike wonder within us that is extraordinary. Children are willing to try anything at a moments notice. The child within you wants to be spontaneous and adventurous. Sadly, spontaneity is easily stifled. Stop being meticulous about planning and organizing all the time. Just follow your heart. Leap into the dance of existence.

Story Telling

Storytelling is conveying events in words, images, and sounds by improvisation or embellishment. Stories or narratives are shared in every culture and in every land as a means of entertainment, education, preservation of culture and in order to instill moral values. Crucial elements of stories and storytelling include plot and characters, as well as the narrative point of view.

Sunscreen

The sun sucks the vitality out of skin turning it leather-like and tough. Sun-skin is old looking and feeling. Always wear sunscreen to protect your skin from the drying rays of the sun and its potential for causing cancer. Soft supple-looking skin is youthful looking and feeling. Use moisturizer if you have dry skin.

Super Foods

Dermatologist Dr. Nicholas Perricone claims that he's found a diet and regimen of supplements and lotions that can make you look younger and live longer. He says his approach can also decrease inflammation in every organ system, improve your metabolism, lift your mood, make your heart resistant to disease, decrease the risk of cancer, improve bone density, repair the skin, rejuvenate your immune system, and possibly help you lose weight. Perricone claims that following his diet and regimen of supplements and lotions helps "reverse the aging process." He says that his diet will make you look younger in as little as three days.

Perricone recommends eating foods with protein, omega-3 fatty acids, and antioxidants. He has identified ten "super-foods", that promote anti-inflammatory activity and reverse aging.

Foods that reverse aging:

1. Acai fruit
2. Allium vegetables: garlic, onions, leeks, scallions, chives, and shallots
3. Barley
4. Green foods like wheatgrass
5. Buckwheat, seeds and grains
6. Beans and lentils
7. Hot pepper
8. Nuts and seeds
9. Sprouts
10. Yogurt and kefir

Supplements

No matter how efficiently and carefully we eat, at times we all
have lows in vitamins and minerals. As we age our food intake
decreases and hence the sufficient proportion of vitamins and
minerals do not reach in body. Certain food restriction also lowers
the intake of vitamins and minerals from natural source. Multi-
vitamin supplements help to keep us healthy, to stave off diseases,
and for youth-extension. Vitamins are anti-oxidants and anti-aging agents that maintain our bodies.

SAMe

European doctors prescribe SAMe (S-adenosylmethionine) for
the therapy of many conditions, including depression, chronic fatigue syndrome, and fibromyalgia. Studies have shown that SAMe
influences the formation of brain chemicals and helps preserve
glutathione, an important antioxidant. Furthermore, SAMe is
involved in the formation of myelin, the white sheath that surrounds nerve cells. Most individuals who take SAMe notice an
increase in concentration, energy, alertness, and well-being. The
influence of SAMe on depression has been tested in numerous
studies. Dozens of clinical studies have demonstrated SAMe's
mood-lifting properties.

Salmon

Salmon is a youth and beauty food because its nutrients play a
key role in keeping the skin's outer layer soft and smooth. The
omega-3s in salmon reduce inflammation on the cellular level that
can cause redness, wrinkles, and loss of firmness. It also fights inflammation, keeping our cells supple, improving circulation, and
helping our brains function optimally.

Sweet Potatoes

Sweet potatoes are filled with the big boost of beauty-enhancing
beta-carotene, a fat-soluble pigment found in many orange vegetables and fruits. It is a powerful antioxidant that protects cells by

destroying the free radicals that can damage them, including skin cells, and cause age-related disorders. The body converts beta-carotene to Vitamin A, which helps keep your skin smooth, so incorporating sweet potatoes into your diet can help you achieve wrinkle-free skin. Beta-carotene also may protect skin from the damage caused by sun exposure.

Swinging

Swinging is sexual activity as a couple with other people that is treated much like any other social activity. Typically, swinging activities occur when a married, or otherwise committed couple, engages in sexual activity with another couple, multiple couples, or a single individual. On these occasions, swingers will often refer to sex as play and sex partners as playmates.

Swinging is a good way for bi-curious women and men to explore their potential bisexuality without becoming involved in the lesbian or gay community where many feel uncomfortable or unwelcome. Swingers claim that this newfound independence from the marriage allows both partners more freedom from one another and their roles which simultaneously makes them happier with the marriage. Due to the very intimate nature of what each partner is doing with other people, good communication is key if the marriage is to survive swinging.

> **Men do not quit playing because they grow old; they grow old because they quit playing.**
>
> ~Oliver Wendell Holmes

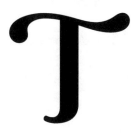

Tea

Tea is the most commonly consumed beverage in the world after water. Black, green, white, and oolong teas derive their leaves from a warm-weather evergreen tree known as *Camellia sinensis*. Leaves from this tree contain polyphenols. The more processing tea leaves undergo, the darker they turn. Green tea and white tea are the least processed tea. Herbal tea is not derived from the leaves of the Camellia plant and so does not have the particular health-promoting properties. Actually, most herbal teas are *not* tea at all.

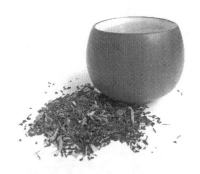

Studies have found that tea drinkers have lower blood pressure and may have lower cholesterol. Black tea seems to lower "bad" cholesterol. Drinking tea might delay

Tea has anti-aging benefits.

Alzheimer's Disease. One researcher found anti-aging benefits when green tea polyphenols were applied directly to skin. It protected the skin by absorbing ultraviolet light and eliminating free radicals.

Testosterone

The hormonal stimulus for sex drive in both men and women is testosterone, which declines with advancing age in both sexes. Testosterone plays an important role in maintaining muscle mass and strength and bone density. Testosterone replacement in males is increasingly used to correct low levels due to disease or aging. The hormone is often administered to aging men and women as a topical cream, but oral testosterone supplements and injectable forms are also available.

Dr. Daniel Amin says that a cranky mood is an indication of low testosterone level in men. He claims to have improved marriages with testosterone therapy. Men over 50 who complain of depression, tiredness, loss of sexual desire, impotence, or muscle weakness may be treated with bioidentical testosterone with good results.

Think Positive

Self-talk is the endless stream of thoughts that run through your head every day, which can be positive or negative. When your self-talk is mostly negative, your outlook on life is more likely pessimistic. The key is to change the way that you talk to yourself. If your thoughts are mostly positive, you're likely an optimist, which will translate into a longer happier, healthier life.

Have you noticed that some older adults continue to feel good and stay active well into their senior years, while others appear to age rapidly and experience increased health problems? Positive thinking plays a significant role in extending youthfulness.

An University of Texas Medical School study said but people who scored high on positive affect or positive thinking were significantly less likely to become frail. The Mayo Clinic reports that positive thinking helps with stress management and can improve health. Health benefits that positive thinking may provide include increased life span, lower rates of depression, lower levels of distress, greater resistance to the common cold, better psychological and physical well-being, reduced risk of death from cardiovascular disease and better coping skills during hardships and times of stress.

Think positive about aging. How you perceive aging affects how long you will live. A Yale study showed that positive perceptions of aging extended lifespan by as much as seven and a half years. Positive views of aging seemed to infuse the will to live, making them more resilient to illness and more proactive in taking care of themselves. Interestingly the study found that positive attitudes about aging increased life more than every other factor they examined—low blood pressure and cholesterol, healthy weight, regular exercise—only not smoking had a more significant impact upon longevity.

Thyroxine

The thyroid gland secretes the hormone thyroxine, which keeps all bodily functions occurring at the correct rate. Skin, bowel activity, muscle, heart rate and other organs are all regulated by thyroxine. Too much thyroxine and the cells in body will be forced to work faster, quickening heart rate, increasing sweat production and raising body temperature. Too little thyroxine and body cells will slow down, resulting in a wide range of symptoms including tiredness, lack of concentration, memory problems, weight gain and low energy levels.

Thyroid deficiency can cause hair loss to fibromyalgia, a common painful musculoskeletal condition. Some of the symptoms of hypothyroidism include fatigue, chilliness, constipation, forgetfulness, muscle cramps, hair loss, depression, sleep disorders, cold hands and feet, dry skin, thinning hair, and weight gain.

Hypothyroidism has been dubbed "the under-diagnosed epidemic". Thyroid testing is often overlooked, resulting in many of us not getting the right thyroid treatment. According to some estimates, as many as fifteen to twenty percent of women over the age of 60 would benefit from thyroid supplements, yet they are not being diagnosed. If you are over 40 years of age and want to slow the aging process, just a small regular whole thyroid supplement can raise energy levels, improve bowel function and improve clear thinking. If you are over 50, you should ask your doctor for a Thyroid Stimulating Hormone (TSH) test at least once every five years—or more often if you have symptoms.

Tryptophan

Often called "nature's prozac" or "nature's serotonin solution", tryptophan (or L-Tryptophan) is an amino acid precursor to serotonin that tends to make people feel good. It is one of the twenty standard amino acids and an essential amino acid in the human diet. Because tryptophan must compete with other amino acids to get into the brain, it can be difficult to maintain adequate levels. Lack of tryptophan can cause or exacerbate depression.

5-HTP is a metabolite of L-Tryptophan and an immediate precursor to serotonin and unlike tryptophan it easily crosses the blood-brain barrier. Its antidepressant effect are more consistent than those reached with tryptophan.

Many people find tryptophan to be a safe and reasonably effective sleep aid, due to its ability to increase brain levels of the calming neurotransmitter serotonin. Tryptophan is found in chocolate, oats, durians, mangoes, dried dates, milk, yogurt, cottage cheese, red meat, eggs, fish, poultry, sesame, chickpeas, sunflower seeds, pumpkin seeds, spirulina, and peanuts.

Turmeric

Turmeric is one of nature's most powerful healers. The active ingredient in turmeric is curcumin. Tumeric has been used for over 2500 years in India. Long known for its anti-inflammatory properties, researchers now believe that most chronic and life-threatening diseases, including those that we commonly think of as accompanying the aging process, are linked to chronic inflammation. Recent research has revealed that turmeric is a natural wonder, proving beneficial in the treatment of many different health conditions from cancer to Alzheimer's disease. Turmeric has also been shown to be a mild anti-bacterial and anti-fungal agent.

Tomatoes

Tomatoes are a beauty food because they are packed with the anti-aging antioxidant lycopene, the bright red carotenoid pigment that gives tomatoes, watermelons, and pink grapefruit their distinctive color. Lycopene is thought to have the highest antioxidant activity of all the carotenoids. Because of its antioxidant effects, lycopene may help protect against cardiovascular disease, cancer, macular degeneration, and possibly other diseases, such as diabetes and osteoporosis.

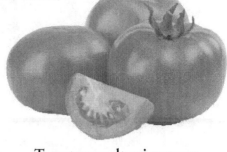

The lycopene in tomatoes is actually more easily absorbed by the body after it is processed into juice, sauce, ketchup, or canned

Tomatoes melt aging away.

tomato puree. Ounce for ounce, the greatest source is canned tomato paste. It's a great staple to keep in your pantry to add to soups or stews for an antioxidant boost.

> I don't believe one grows older. I
> think that what happens early on in
> life is that at a certain age one stands
> still and stagnates.
>
> ~T.S. Eliot

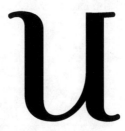

Unicorn

A unicorn is a mythological creature that has have held a sense of mystery and promise of untold adventures. Because of the unicorn's purity, its horn, sometimes called an "ulicorn", was considered magical and became a popular ingredient in medieval medicines. Its presence was considered a strong protection against poison in food, and when worn in jewelry protected the wearer from evil.

Unicorns represent truth, purity, innocence, trust, strength and courage. Believe in unicorns. Thinking about beauty has a soothing effect on the psychie and boosts the immune system. Unicorns are beautiful. A unicorn saved Harry Potter from He-Who-Cannot-Be-Named. Kids find it easy to believe in mysteries and create fantasies. Exercise your child brain, believe in unicorns. Doing so will bring you long life and good health.

"Do you know, I always thought unicorns were fabulous monsters, too? I never saw one alive before!" "Well, now that we have seen each other," said the unicorn, "if you'll believe in me, I'll believe in you."

--Lewis Carroll
Through the Looking Glass

Unicycle

It's cool to be up on one wheel. Unicycling gets your juices flowing and your brain secreting dopamine and serotonin, the feel-good hormones because its fun and gives you a good exercise workout. When unicycling you get a lot of exercise because you are always pedaling. Riding is a low-impact activity, so it puts less stress on your legs than when jogging. Unicycle cruising speed is 8-9 miles an hour on a standard 24" unicycle, which is fast enough to get you around town.

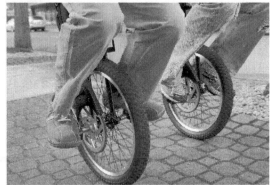

Unicycling gets feel-good hormones flowing.

Unicycling is constantly challenging. Rising to challenges keep us young. After you learn to ride forward on your unicycle, you can learn to ride backwards. Then you can learn to ride one-footed. Learning causes the brain to grow and growing brain is a young brain. Keep your brain growing. Ride a unicycle. Then you can join the circus if you ever lose your job or simply drop out. Good to have a plan!

Ukulele

The ukulele is a small guitar-like instrument brought to Hawaii by Portuguese immigrants. It's fairly easy to learn to play. Take up the uke! With just a few chords and strumming techniques you can bring the joy of music to any event. Music makes us feel good. Singing with friends builds bonds and ups the positive impact of socializing on our psychies. Take up the ukulele and be the life of the party. How much fun is that?

It's sad to grow old, but nice to ripen.

~Brigitte Bardot

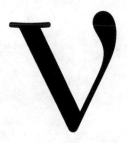

Viagra®

Viagra®—sildenafil—is used to treat erectile dysfunction— impotence—in men. Another brand of sildenafil is Revatio®, which is used to treat pulmonary arterial hypertension and improve exercise capacity in men and women.

Sildenafil's use is now standard treatment for erectile dysfunction in all settings, including diabetes and usually improves sexual function in men. The penis uses pressurized blood to get rigid. When a man becomes aroused, the arteries leading into the penis open up so that pressurized blood can enter the penis quickly. The veins leaving the penis constrict. Pressurized blood is trapped in the *corpora cavernosa*, and this blood causes the penis to elongate and stiffen. The penis is erect. If the arteries leading to the penis don't open up properly, it is difficult or impossible for a man to become erect. Viagra® relaxes the arterial wall, leading to decreased pulmonary arterial resistance and pressure. Studies on the effects of Viagra® when used recreationally are limited, but suggest that it has little effect when used by those not suffering from erectile dysfunction.

Vinpocetine

Vinpocetine is a nootropic or "smart drug", extracted from periwinkle used throughout the world to treat brain aging. The scientific literature provides persuasive evidence that this plant extract can improve memory and cognitive function. Normal aging results in a reduction of blood flow to the brain and a decrease in the metabolic activity of brain cells. The biological actions of vinpocetine initially showed that it enhances circulation and oxygen utilization in the brain, increases tolerance of the brain towards diminished blood flow, and inhibits abnormal platelet aggregation that can interfere with circulation or cause a stroke.

Visualize

Visualization is a powerful manifestation tool. Everything that was ever created by humans began as a concept or mental picture. Many successful athletes visualize themselves being victorious, they actually feel, taste and even smell victory.

Visualization is using the Law of Attraction for conscious creation. According to the law of attraction you will attract into your life what you focus on. With visualization and the use of affirmations you can attract anything you want. If you create a mental image or movie of success, you will be successful. Visualization is essentially the process of guided imagery meditation. Get yourself into a deeply-relaxed state and then use your mind to create positive images of something you want to have, or be. Create a mental image or movie of something and play it over and over.

The first step is to determine a plan or desire to be fulfilled. Sit in a relaxed position, close your eyes, and breathe slowly and deeply. Enjoy the feeling of your breath going in and out slowly and deeply. In your mind *see* yourself at the time when your desire is achieved or your plan is accomplished. By *seeing yourself in the goal state* your desire or picture is "burned" into your unconscious.

Use the magic of visualization to imagine see yourself youthful and full of energy. Soon you will find yourself to be curiously reinvigorated.

Vitamin A—Beta-Carotene

Vitamin A is the anti-infection vitamin and is important in the body's defense system. European cancer specialist, Dr. Hans Neiper recommends using high doses of beta-carotene—especially in the form of carrot juice. Beta-carotene is necessary for skin, hair and nails. It slows aging of the face.

Vitamin B-1—Thiamin

Thiamin is necessary for energy production and optimal nerve transmission. It assists in fatty-acid formation of neurons, in the synthesis of acetylcholine, a neurotransmitter, and helps counteract the aging effects of cigarette smoke and alcohol. It is helpful in prevention of psychiatric and neurological disorders. Thiamin is found in carbohydrate-rich foods, including beans, peas, lentils, raw nuts, whole grains, and yogurt.

Vitamin B-2—Riboflavin

Riboflavin is important for body growth and red blood cell production and helps in releasing energy from carbohydrates. Riboflavin is water soluble, which means it is not stored in the body and must be replenished everyday. Riboflavin is found in lean meats, eggs, legumes, nuts, green leafy vegetables, dairy products, and milk.

Vitamin B-3—Niacin

Niacin combats depression, insomnia, anxiety and fatigue Austrian scientists showed that niacin niacin's influence of dopamine production was successful in treating Parkinson's patients and reduced in disease-related depressive symptoms. It also dilates blood vessels. Taken over the course of several years, it reduces the chance for cardiovascular problems and senility.

Vitamin B-5—Pantothenic

Pantothenic acid, often called the "anti-stress" vitamin, is important for growth, reproduction and normal physiological function. Pantothenic acid helps change carbohydrates and glucose, or sugar, into energy, helps breakdown fats and proteins, and helps keep the body's nervous system running and healthy. It protects arteries against cholesterol damage, stimulates cells of the immune system, helps to form red blood cells, antibodies, lipids, neurotransmitters, hormones and antibodies.

Like the rest of the B vitamins, pantothenic acid is water soluble and cannot be stored in the body. Pantothenic acid is found in avocados, eggs, milk, beef, legumes, salmon, grains, mushrooms, broccoli, collard greens and other fresh vegetables. It can be manufactured in the intestine.

Vitamin B-6—Pyridoxine

Pyridoxine plays a vital role in the activities of many enzymes essential for the breakdown and use of proteins, carbohydrates and fats from food and for the release of stored carbohydrates for energy. It is involved in the production of red blood cells and antibodies and in the maintenance of a healthy skin and healthy digestion. B-6 increases T-cells, T-helper cells, and antibodies and is important for normal function of the nervous system and several hormones. It boosts immune system, reduces homocysteine in blood vessels, which leads to greater protection against heart attacks and disease. Pyridoxine helps prevent age-related memory decline and aides in the transport and metabolism of amino acids used by the brain to build neurotransmitters.

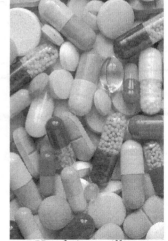

Pyridoxine is found in liver, chicken, wholemeal cereals, wheat-germ and eggs are particularly rich sources. Bananas, avocados and pota-toes also contain pyridoxine

Vitamin B-9—Folic Acid

Folate is necessary for the production and maintenance of new cells. It is especially important during periods of rapid cell division and growth such

Youth in a pill!!!

as infancy and pregnancy and to prevent neurological damage
during early fetal development. It reduces risk of stroke and may
help prevent cancer because of its role in the synthesis, repair,
and functioning of DNA, and a deficiency of folate may result
in damage to DNA that may lead to cancer. In a study of people
over 50, short-term memory, mental agility, and verbal fluency all
improved among those subjects who took 800 micrograms of folic
acid daily, twice the current RDA, than those who took placebo.

Vitamin B-12—Cobalamin

Cobalamin functions as a methyl donor and works with folic acid
in the synthesis of DNA and red blood cells. It is important in
maintaining the health of the insulation sheath—myelin sheath—
that surrounds nerve cells. Cobalamin helps to increase oxygen
delivery to the brain. Cobalamin reverses "pseudo-senility," a
condition mimicking dementia or Alzheimer's, but stems from
a B-12 deficiency. With age, the stomach becomes less able to
absorb B-12 and levels drop. Supplementing what one eats can
dramatically raise levels and mental functioning.

Vitamin C—Ascorbic Acid

Vitamin C, also known as ascorbic acid, calcium ascorbate, and
sodium ascorbate, is a water-soluble vitamin necessary for normal
growth and development. It may be the single more important
vitamin for the immune system and is famous for battling the
common cold.

Vitamin C is used in manufacturing the neurotransmitter,
norepinephrine. Neurotransmitters are critical to brain function
and are known to affect mood. It reduces high blood pressure and
detrimental LDL cholesterol; increases positive HDL cholesterol,
vitamin E, and glutatione levels; cleans and strengthens blood
vessel walls; stops oxidative damage to eyes, gum tissues, and male
sperm; and provides powerful protection against cancer.

Ascorbic acid is an antioxidant that stops free radical chain
reactions within watery part of tissues and is required for the synthesis of neurotransmitters acetylcholine and norepinphrine.

Green peppers, citrus fruits and juices, strawberries, tomatoes, broccoli, turnip greens and other leafy greens, sweet and white potatoes, and cantaloupe are sources of Vitamin C.

Vitamin D

Vitamin D is a fat-soluble vitamin essential for promoting calcium absorption in the gut and maintaining adequate serum calcium and phosphate concentrations to enable normal mineralization of bone and prevent hypocalcemic tetany. It is also needed for bone growth and bone remodeling by osteoblasts and osteoclasts. Vitamin D plays an important role in the modulation of neuromuscular and immune function and reduction of inflammation.

A growing body of research suggests that Vitamin D might play some role in the prevention and treatment of type 1 and type 2 diabetes, hypertension, glucose intolerance, multiple sclerosis, and other medical conditions. Most people meet their Vitamin D needs through exposure to sunlight. The flesh of fish (such as salmon, tuna, and mackerel) and fish liver oils are among the best sources

Vitamin E

Acting in conjunction with vitamins A and C and selenium, Vitamin E is an antioxidant and scavenger of toxic free radicals. Vitamin E reduces detrimental LDL cholesterol, which keeps arteries from clogging; prevents heart attacks, strokes; rejuvenates immunity and blocks cancer cell growth; protects against degenerative brain diseases; and relieves arthritis and fights cataracts.

You're never too old to become younger.

—Mae West

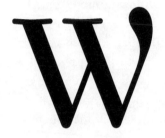

Walk

Walking reduces the risk of many diseases—from heart attack to hip fracture. Melbourne research showed that walking improves memory and can protect from the ravages of dementia. Walking improves lower body strength, maintains mobility and helps lessen cognitive decline.

Walk on a cobblestone path. Scientists believe that walking on uneven surfaces like cobblestones improves the vestibular system of the inner ear, which plays a central role in balance and equilibrium.

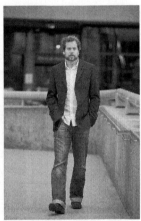

Walking melts the years away.

Walnuts

Smooth skin tone, healthy hair, vibrant eyes, and strong bones can all be attributed to nutrients found in walnuts. Walnuts contain a significant amount of beauty-enhancing omega-3 fatty acids, plus they provide Vitamin E, a fat-soluble antioxidant that protects cells from free-radical damage and is associated with beautiful skin.

Research has revealed that eating just four walnuts a day for three weeks significantly increases blood levels not only of alpha-linolenic acid, the essential omega-3 fatty acid, but also of its longer chain derivative, eicosapentaenoic acid. Walnuts are a fantastic way to add nutrients, taste, and crunch to your diet. You can eat them by themselves or throw a handful into your cereal, salad, or stir-fry.

Water

Water is essential for hydration of the skin, muscles, circulation, and all organs in the body. Frequent drinks of good water is crucial. Enjoy six to eight glasses of pure water daily in addition to other liquids and watery foods. Many people's health problems and anti-aging would improve if they would just drink more good water.

Watermelon

The flesh and seeds of the watermelon are both nutritious. When blended together in a food processor they make a youth-promoting delicious juice. The flesh contain Vitamin A, B and C; the seeds contain selenium, essential fats, zinc and vitamin E, all of which help against free radical damage to keep us young and sassy.

Watermelon Blueberry Banana Split

2 large bananas

8 watermelon "scoops"—watermelon balls created with an ice cream scoop

2 cups fresh blueberries

½ cup low-fat vanilla yogurt

½ cup low-fat granola

Peel bananas and cut in half crosswise, then cut each piece in half lengthwise. For each serving lay 2 banana pieces against the sides of a shallow dish. Place a watermelon scoop at each

end of the dish. Fill the center space with blueberries. Stir
yogurt until smooth and spoon over watermelon scoops.
Sprinkle with granola. 4 servings
                    —Centers for Disease Control and Prevention

Wheatgrass

Wheatgrass is the young grass of the wheat plant, *Triticum
aestivum*, that has been freshly juiced. Wheatgrass has regenerative
powers and an ability to boost the immune system. It is highly
nutritious, containing most of the vitamins and minerals needed
for human maintenance, including complete protein with about
30 enzymes and approximately seventy percent chlorophyll. It
is an excellent source of calcium, iron, magnesium, phosphorus,
potassium, sodium, sulphur, cobalt, and zinc.

The high chlorophyll content of wheatgrass juice causes
increased hemoglobin production in the body, which in turn
increases the oxygen carrying capabilities of the blood. The
increased capability of the blood to carry oxygen has a number
of health benefits including purification of the blood, improving blood sugar disorders, helping combat toxins such as carbon
monoxide and other traffic pollutants, cigarette smoke and heavy
metals that can get into the blood.

Whole Grains

Whole grains provide soluble fiber to help lower blood cholesterol
levels, and also have phytonutrient content equal to any fruit or
vegetable. Whole grain is a diet-friendly food. Whole grains offer
protection against diabetes, heart disease, stroke, colon cancer, high
blood pressure, and gum disease. These benefits are tied to the array
of vitamins, minerals, plant chemicals, and again, fiber that work
together to promote health. Eat whole grain breads and cereals.
Your body will thank you.

Wonder

We live in a true Alice-in-Wonderland-like Universe. Awesome
and unfathomable. Yet, we become complacent so that the awesome

> Youthfulness is connected to the ability to see things new for the first time. So if your eyes still look at life with wonder, then you will seem young, even though you may not be chronologically young.
>
> —Goldie Hawn

becomes commonplace. A beautiful rose emerges from the earth— amazing! But we don't notice the magic. We become blind. Our eyes see but *we don't see*. We lose ability to wonder because we're too sophisticated, or too busy, or too absorbed. We grow old. We lose ability to find rapt attention or astonishment at something awesomely mysterious. We forget to appreciate the miracle of existence. So we grow old.

To regain child-like wonder is the greatest youth elixir. Take every opportunity to experience something as though coming in contact with it for the first time. Purposefully express wonder at the world, and take every opportunity to experience something new. Look for opportunities to say, "WOW!"

Have you not been paying attention?
Have you not been listening?
Haven't you heard these stories all your life?
Don't you understand the foundation of all things?
God sits high above the round ball of earth.
The people look like mere ants.
He stretches out the skies like a canvas—
yes, like a tent canvas to live under.
He ignores what all the princes say and do.
The rulers of the earth count for nothing.
Princes and rulers don't amount to much.
Like seeds barely rooted, just sprouted,
They shrivel when God blows on them.
Like flecks of chaff, they're gone with the wind.
Have you not been paying attention?
Have you not been listening?
Haven't you heard these stories all your life?
—Isaiah 40: 21-24

Worry Beads

Worry beads, traditionally known as "Komboloi", are a string of beads for fingering in times of worry, boredom, or tension. They help you to stay calm when dealing with the worries, anxiety and stress that seem to plague many of us daily. Unlike other forms of prayer beads, the worry beads do not have religious significance. They are merely seen as an instrument of relaxation and stress management.

Wrinkle Treatments

Wrinkles are a natural part of aging. With age, skin gets thinner, drier and less elastic, becoming less able to protect itself from damage. As a result, wrinkles, lines and creases form in the skin. Sun exposure and smoking accelerate skin aging and wrinkle formation.

Wrinkle treatments include topical retinoids. Derived from Vitamin A, retinoids reduce fine wrinkles, splotchy pigmentation and skin roughness. retinol, alpha hydroxy acids, kinetin, coenzyme Q10, copper peptides and antioxidants may result

> **Cheerfulness and contentment are great beautifiers and are famous preservers of youthful looks.**
> —Eschylus

in slight to modest improvements in wrinkles. Surgical procedures include dermabrasion, a procedure that consists of sanding down (planing) the surface layer of the skin with a rapidly rotating brush. The planing removes the skin surface and a new layer of skin grows in its place. Another method is laser treatments. In ablative (wounding) laser resurfacing, a laser beam destroys the outer layer of skin (epidermis) and heats the underlying skin (dermis), which stimulates the growth of new collagen fibers. As the wound heals, new skin forms that's smoother and tighter.

Chemical peel is a popular treatment. A doctor applies an acid to the affected areas, which burns the outer layer of the skin. With medium-depth peels, the entire epidermis and a small portion of the dermis are removed. New skin forms to take its place. The new skin is usually smoother and less wrinkled than the old skin. Another treatment is Botox, which when injected in small doses into specific muscles blocks the chemical signals that cause muscles to contract. When the muscles can't tighten, the skin flattens and appears smoother and less wrinkled. Botox works well on frown lines between the eyebrows and across the forehead, and crow's-feet at the corners of the eyes.

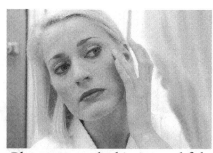

Plump, smooth skin is youthful.

Another treatment is soft tissue fillers, which include fat, collagen and hyaluronic acid is injected into deeper wrinkles on the face. They plump and smooth out wrinkles and furrows and give the skin more volume.

Acting childish seems to come naturally, but acting like an adult, no
matter how old we are, just doesn't
come easy to us.

—Lily Tomlin

Xenodochial

Xenodochial is extending hospitality and kindliness to strangers, especially foreigners. Youth tends to be open to the new and different. They love to travel and experience cultures of people of different nations. Getting to know strangers expands our world and keep us young in spirit.

Xylomancy

Xylomancy is a form of divination that is practiced by the Slavs. The divination is done by interpreting the shape and position of dry pieces of wood found in one`s path. These are considered Omens. Divination, practice of foreseeing future events or obtaining secret knowledge through communication with divine sources and through omens, oracles, signs, and portents. It is based on the belief in revelations offered to humans by the gods and in extra-rational forms of knowledge; it attempts to make known those things that neither reason nor science can discover.

> **You don't stop laughing because you grow old;**
> **You grow old because you stop laughing.**
>
> —Michael Pritchard

Y

Yachting

Imagine the wind in your face and the soothing sounds of water on the bow caressing your senses gently. The sound of the ocean, dolphins, the calls of birds, and the waves lapping against the hull are the sounds used for meditation and massage to promote stress relief and total relaxation. Yachting is healthy and youth-enhancing. Hoisting sails and trimming them, balancing on a moving platform is a gentle form of exercise. It's fun, too. You might even quit your job and sail the world—but stay away from the pirates, who are no fun at all.

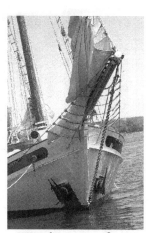

Wind in your face.

Yodel

Yodeling is singing an extended note rapidly and repeatedly with changes in pitch from the chest register to the falsetto making a high-low-high-low sound. Yodeling is actually good for you because offers both physical and mental health benefits. It opens up the lungs, relieves stress, awakens the soul and opens you up for the possibility of the day. Like yoga, the secret to a good yodel is in mastery of the breathing, which aids in releasing stress and calming nerves.

The best places for Alpine-style yodeling are those with an echo such as a mountain range. Lakes, rocky gorges, anywhere with a distant rock face, between office buildings, or down a long hallway are good places to practice yodeling. Take up yodeling. Certificate courses in "yodel-ology" are available via the Internet.

Yoga And Meditation

Yoga is a combination of breathing and body postures that increases blood circulation. Yoga strengthens muscles and regulates the flow of oxygen in the system. Yoga must be practiced regularly to reap the long-term effects. Yoga keeps the body fit and energy level high thus suppressing aging. Yoga helps in maintaining weight by burning fat and increases metabolic rate to certain extent. It involves no external application or intake of any medicine. Yoga is the most simple and natural way to stay fit physically and mentally.

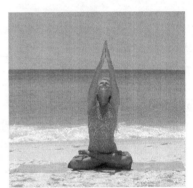

Rejuvenate mind and body.

Yogurt

Soviet Georgia is claimed to have more centenarians per capita than any other country. Many claim that the secret of their long lives is yogurt, which they eat with nearly every meal. While the age-defying powers of yogurt have not been proven scientifically, yogurt is rich in calcium, which helps stave off osteoporosis and contains "good bacteria" that help maintain intestinal health. Calcium promotes strong bones, beautiful nails, good posture, and a beautiful smile. Eight ounces of yogurt has two grams of zinc, which is beneficial for the skin. At about 150 calories per cup, plain low-fat yogurt is a slimming treat. Enjoy a cup of yogurt and make sure to hold up your little finger while eating it so those watching know that you, too, are cultured.

Yohimbe

Yohimbe is an evergreen tree that grows in western Africa in Nigeria, Cameroon, the Congo and Gabon. An alkaloid derived from yohimbe is used in conventional drugs for male impotence and yohimbe has become a prominent, if controversial, herb for promoting sexual desire and performance. The herb does have definite effects on aspects of sexual performance—ability to increase blood flow to the penis and cause "erectile stimulation." Yohimbe is approved by the FDA for treatment of male impotence. Oh yeah!

A man is not old until regrets take the place of dreams.

-John Barrymore

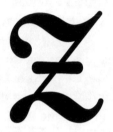

Zest

Zest an enjoyably exciting quality characteristic of youth. Youth lives with gusto, doing everything with zeal and enthusiasm. One of the worst things about aging is the lost of youthful zest for life. How do we get it back? Zest is promoted by first time experiences—learning something new and which causes us to look to the future. Learn new things and try new experiences. You have to stretch yourself. Get out of your comfort zone.

Working to meet important goals and then achieving them provides new experiences, knowledge, skills and a richer future. The joy of accomplishment and the experience of the task itself are the ingredients to that zest for life. Imagine what you want, formulate a plan, then make it happen. That is how as adults we regain our zest for Living. Do things with zest and your life will become more exciting, enjoyable and interesting.

Zen

The Zen way is to return to the beginning. Stop, sit down, look within. Remember where we came from, who we are and where we are headed. Remember to take care of our simple lives as well as the lives of others along the way. Sorrow and joy, anxiety and imperturbability cannot be avoided. However Zen teaches that by not clinging to them we can be free, no longer pulled this way and that.

We create all kinds of goals and drive ourselves crazy to reach them. We measure our progress, compare ourselves to others, judge ourselves relentlessly. This is not the Zen way. In Zen, focus upon each breath, each day, each moment and experience it totally. As you begin to live the Zen way, you develop a new way of knowing and of being in the world. You do not analyze, explain or justify what happens. Rather than try to mold or control our experience, simply make friends with it, become acquainted, and let it instruct you.

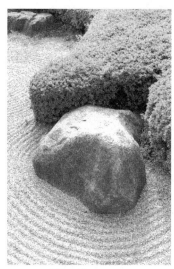

The Zen way.

Central and indispensable to Zen is daily *Zazen* practice. Zazen is a Japanese term consisting of two characters: *za*, "to sit cross-legged," and *zen*, from the Sanscrit dhyana, meaning at once concentration, dynamic stillness, and contemplation. With time and sincere effort in Zazen practice, mind and body, inside and outside, self and other are experienced as one. The condition of effortless concentration, is known as *Samadhi*. By returning to your original nature, you remember how to sit, breathe, eat, play and re-claim the excitement, joy and adventure we felt as children, but lost along the way.

Zany

Zany relates to play and all things fun. It is acting like the buffoon to amuse others. Be silly. Revive your inner child and play, play, play.

Zinc

Zinc citrate rejuvenates the thymus gland, which boosts immune system through T-cell formation. It destroys free radicals and increases albumin and gamma interferon levels. Vegetarians and those on low calorie diets are very susceptible to zinc deficiency. A deficiency of zinc can lead to "psuedo-senility" in elderly people.

Zone

The 'zone' is a place in the mind where time seems to stand still or even disappear. When in the zone movements are fluid and natural, yet effortlessly controlled. Tasks transcend the mundane, reaching a perfection of focus far beyond everyday concentration. When entering the zone, even though the body may be active, the mind has a center of stillness and peace, free of concern.

Think back to your best performance. Did it feel easy or difficult? Whether it was the perfect drive, scoring with ease or running the perfect race, how did it feel? It was easy wasn't it! It took no effort at all and just the act of performing was a joy.

Being in the zone is, in fact, being in a particular kind of trance state. Time doesn't matter. Senses are heightened. Everything feels effortless and good. Often called "Flow", the zone is where we are at our peak productivity.

> **To get back one's youth one has merely to repeat one's follies.**
>
> —Oscar Wilde

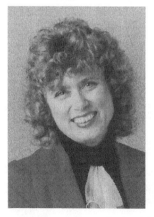

Dr. Beverly Potter's work blends the philosophies of humanistic psychology and Eastern mysticism with principles of behavior psychology to create an inspiring approach to handling the many challenges encountered in today's workplace.

Docpotter earned her Masters of Science in vocational rehabilitation counseling from San Francisco State and her doctorate in counseling psychology from Stanford University. She was a member of the staff development team at Stanford University for nearly twenty years.

Beverly is a dynamic and informative speaker. Her workshops have been sponsored by numerous colleges including San Francisco State Extended Education, DeAnza and Foothill Colleges Short Courses, University of California at Berkeley Extension, as well as corporations such as Hewlett Packard, Cisco Systems, Genentech, Sun Microsystems, Becton-Dickenson and Tap Plastics; government agencies like California Disability Evaluation, Department of Energy, IRS Revenue Officers; and professional associations such as California Continuing Education of the Bar, Design Management Institute, and International Association of Personnel Women. Docpotter's many books are listed in the front. Her website is *docpotter.com*. You can also find her on Twitter, Facebook and elswhere in cyberspace. Please visit.

Ronin Books-for-Independent-Minds

MANAGING YURSELF FOR EXCELLENCE .... Potter MANYOU 12.95 ___
How to become a can-do person.

PREVENTING JOB BURNOUT .... Potter PREJOB 12.95 ___
Workbook: How to renew enthusiasm for work.

HIGH PERFORMANCE GOAL SETTING .... Potter HIGOAL 9.95 ___
How to use intuition to conceive and achieve your dreams.

GET PEAK PERFORMANCE EVERY DAY .... Potter GETPEA 12.95 ___
How to manage like a coach.

FINDING A PATH WITH A HEART .... Potter FINPAT 14..95 ___
How to go from burnout to bliss, principles of self-leading.

BEYOND CONSCIOUSNESS .... Potter BEYCON 14.00 ___
What happens after death. Very comforting for the grieving.

THE WAY OF THE RONIN .... Potter WAYRON 14.95 ___
Maverick career strategies for riding the waves of change at work.

FROM CONFLICT TO COOPERATION .... Potter FROCON 14.95 ___
How to mediate a dispute, step-by-step technique.

MAVERICK AS MASTER IN THE MARKET PLACE .... Potter MAVMAS 9.95 ___
Audio: The way of the office warrior

WORRYWART'S COMPANION .... Potter WORWAR 15.95 ___
21 ways to soothe yourself and worry smart.

DRUG TESTING AT WORK .... Potter & Orfali DRUTES 24.95 ___
A guide for employers.

PASS THE TEST .... Potter & Orfali PASTES 16.95 ___
An employee guide to drug testing.

PRICE & AVAILABILITY
SUBJECT TO CHANGE
WITHOUT NOTICE

Books prices: SUBTOTAL $_____
CA customers add sales tax 9.75% _____
BASIC SHIPPING: (All orders) **$6.00**

PLUS SHIPPING: USA+$1 for each book, Canada+$2 for each book } $_____
Europe+$7 for each book, Pacific+$10 for each book
Books + Tax + Basic + Shipping: TOTAL $_____

Checks payable to **Ronin Publishing**

MC _ Visa _ Exp date _ _ - _ _ card #: _ _ _ _ _ _ _ _ _ _ _ _ _ _ _ _ _ _ (sign) _ _ _ _ _ _ _ _ _

Name_ _

Address _ _ _ _ _ _ _ _ _ _ _ _ _ City _ _ _ _ _ _ _ _ _ _ _ _ _ State _ _ _ ZIP _ _ _ _ _.

☞ Call for our FREE catalog. On-line catalog-> www.roninpub.com
Go to amazon.com or order through your independent bookstore.
Ask your library to add Docpotter's books to their collection.

✍ **Ronin Books-By-Phone • Box 22900 Oakland CA 94609**
Stores & Distributors — Call for Wholesale info and catalog